Intelligent Drugs: How AI is Transforming Healthcare

Philippe Moingeon

Intelligent Drugs: How AI is Transforming Healthcare

Springer

Philippe Moingeon
Paris-Saclay University
Orsay, Essonne, France

ISBN 978-3-031-91667-0 ISBN 978-3-031-91668-7 (eBook)
https://doi.org/10.1007/978-3-031-91668-7

Translation from the French language edition: "L'intelligence artificielle au service de la santé" by Philippe Moingeon, © DeBoeck 2024. Published by DeBoeck. All Rights Reserved.

The original submitted manuscript has been translated into English. The translation was done using artificial intelligence. A subsequent revision was performed by the author(s) to further refine the work and to ensure that the translation is appropriate concerning content and scientific correctness. It may, however, read stylistically different from a conventional translation.

This Springer imprint is published by the registered company Springer Nature Switzerland AG
The registered company address is: Gewerbestrasse 11, 6330 Cham, Switzerland

Foreword

The use of artificial intelligence has taken on considerable importance in all areas of science, particularly in medical and pharmaceutical sciences. The discovery of new drugs can indeed benefit from artificial intelligence for the discovery of new therapeutic targets, the selection of the most effective molecules thanks to combinatorial chemistry, the orientation of pharmacological and toxicological tests at the preclinical level as well as the optimized conduct of clinical trials. It also allows the identification of possible drug interactions that the human mind could not highlight due to the very large amount of data available. Using artificial intelligence to design and develop faster, more effective, and less toxic drugs represents a highly multidisciplinary approach, combining mathematics with chemistry, molecular and cellular biology, pharmacology, and toxicology.

This approach has become essential today due to the increasing number of data resulting from the acceleration of open science. This now encourages researchers worldwide to publish their work in open access journals, associating the raw data of their research, disseminated online for free, and freely. Databases are therefore expected to multiply exponentially over the decade; they contain new therapeutic leads for designing intelligent drugs for more personalized medicine. Artificial intelligence is indeed capable of taking into account the very great biological diversity of patients in order to identify the subgroup of patients likely to respond better to a treatment with a minimum of side effects. The sequencing of the human genome as well as molecular profiling and diagnostic technologies provide a mass of useful data, which the human brain would however take a long time to process. Computer-simulated clinical studies can also be considered before any clinical trial. At the preclinical level, artificial intelligence contributes to accelerating the discovery of new drugs by better orienting research paths and also reducing the number of animals to be used in pharmacological and toxicological tests, before moving on to human clinical trials. New frontiers of science can now be explored to better understand certain complex pathophysiological mechanisms at the origin of serious diseases that we still know little about, particularly in the field of oncology, neuroscience, and immune diseases. The use of algorithms also allows innovation through breakthrough and less conventional therapeutic approaches. Among others, synthetic biology, the use of stem cells for organ reconstruction or chimeric antigen receptor T cells for cancer immunotherapy, as well as the use of nanotechnologies to deliver the drug at the right time and the right place in the body, or to develop molecular-scale imaging and diagnostic methods.

Easy to read by specialists as well as non-specialists, this book should interest a wide audience of students, academic and industrial researchers, health professionals, doctors and pharmacists, but also engineers, scientists, and mathematicians interested in biomedical sciences.

A senior executive in pharmaceutical industry research, Philippe Moingeon holds a PhD in Immunology and an MBA in technology management. He is perfectly qualified to address all aspects, both scientific, economic, and societal, related to the use of artificial intelligence to discover innovative drugs. He has created a particularly active working group on this subject at the National Academy of Pharmacy, and he has set up the first "Artificial Intelligence and Drug Science" course as well as a certifying diploma on AI in health at the University of Paris-Saclay. Readers will certainly be pleased to benefit from his excellent expertise on this current scientific and societal topic.

Patrick COUVREUR, Emeritus Professor at University of Paris-Saclay, Member of the Academy of Sciences and Honorary President of the French Academy of Pharmacy, Former Professor at the Collège de France.

Patrick Couvreur

Preface

The Emergence of Intelligent Drugs

The resolution of the COVID-19 pandemic required an unprecedented revolution in how we design, test, and regulate new drugs. This shared experience has particularly highlighted the synergy between biotechnologies and artificial intelligence (AI). At the same time, unfounded fears toward proven effective vaccines, but also mistrust toward the pharmaceutical industry—despite demonstrating its societal utility to the world—have revealed a deep lack of knowledge of the drug universe in the general population.

As an immunologist, I have been exploring for more than 7 years the interest of AI in designing drugs against diseases of the immune system. Convinced of its revolutionary potential in this field, I founded a think tank within the French Academy of Pharmacy, as well as a specialized course at the University Paris-Saclay to introduce both students, academic and industrial researchers, and health professionals to the multiple contributions of these new technologies in the drug universe. It also seemed necessary to inform the general public about this revolution that concerns—or will concern—each of us during our life, given the dramatic changes underway. My wish here is to make the current field of drugs more understandable, by clearly explaining its anticipated advancements and challenges, in light of the profound transformations that are coming.

Terms such as *big data*, artificial neural networks, machine learning, and generative AI are now part of our daily life, illustrating the intrusion of these new technologies, especially in the field of health. Today, new drugs are designed by computer, allowing to choose from billions of virtual molecules those that possess the desired properties. Even before chemists synthesize selected drug candidates, their effectiveness can be studied on just as virtual patients! Far from a science fiction scenario, these predictive models are now becoming commonly used by researchers in the pharmaceutical industry.

This profound change is not the result of chance, it is the culmination of continuous advances in scientific knowledge and technologies over half a century. However, the importance of changes underway has only truly been evident through a series of very recent developments. In 2015, a new AI method called "deep learning" allowed the creation of very efficient predictive algorithms, with many applications in the medical field. As early as 2017, Stanford University trained artificial neural networks to identify skin cancers with a reliability comparable to that of the most experienced dermatologists. The same year, the American regulatory agency *Food and Drug Administration* (FDA) granted for the first time a market authorization for drugs targeting specific DNA mutations in tumors, regardless of the organ affected. These achievements, seemingly disparate, reflect converging forces that are profoundly transforming drug research and medicine. They indeed illustrate the promise of considerable synergies between AI and drug sciences, to accelerate innovation and allow the design of "intelligent" drugs optimally adapted to the characteristics of patients, whatever their diseases.

To account for this exciting evolution, we will first draw lessons from the health crisis related to COVID-19 and its resolution thanks to effective vaccines developed in record time. We will further discuss an innovation now exponential, for the benefit of patients, made possible by the conjunction of technologies providing health data in gigantic quantity, exploited with the AI to design novel therapeutic approaches based on biotechnologies and other disruptive drug modalities.

In a second part, we will describe the different faces of this transformation by AI of the drug life cycle. These cover the computer design of drug candidates to best meet the needs of patients, the prediction of their pharmacological properties and their evaluation using virtual patients or digital twins. The contributions will also be significant on the production and dispensation of the drug, materialized by an evolution toward a pharmaceutical industry 4.0 and an "intelligent" hospital of the future.

A third part will be devoted to the medium-term consequences for the patient and for medicine of these upheavals induced by AI. A new medicine that we will call "computational precision medicine" now integrates an unprecedented level of knowledge of the characteristics of each patient, but also of existing or potential virtual drugs, to allow a more personalized treatment. This medicine will offer in the coming years many innovative drugs, increasingly effective and safer against the majority of diseases. It will be predictive of health risks not yet declared and will propose drugs to prevent diseases, or to treat them very early. Beyond, smart drugs and medical devices will allow those who wish to enhance the performance of their bodies, boost their intelligence, and even slow down aging, with the promise of a significant increase in healthy life expectancy.

Finally, we will consider the societal implications of this revolution in medicine powered by AI in the coming decades. Undoubtedly, these will be substantial and multidimensional, requiring a radical overhaul of health systems to ensure the management of an unprecedented wave of innovative drugs. But also protection of the privacy of personal health data, as well as the development of an AI ethics concerned with the human to accompany technological innovation in health. The revolution associated with intelligent drugs has already been initiated, beyond doubt; it will only make sense if it eventually benefits all of humanity.

Orsay, France Philippe Moingeon

Competing Interests The author has no competing interests to declare that are relevant to the content of this manuscript.

Contents

About the Author

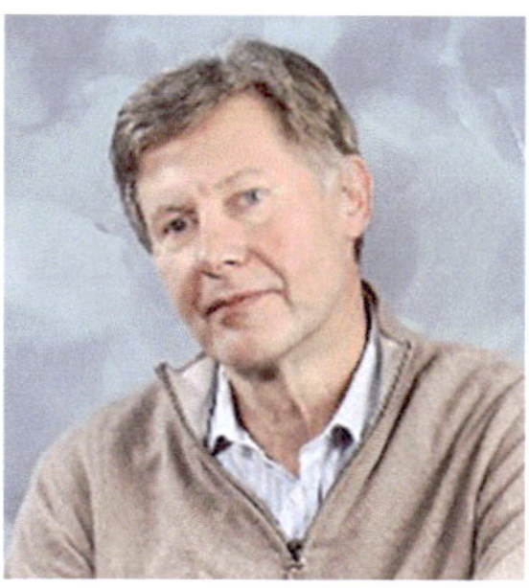

Philippe Moingeon is an immunologist, former researcher, and Assistant Professor at Harvard Medical School (Boston, USA), and Professor in AI and Health at Paris-Saclay University. He is a member of the French Academy of Pharmacy, and an expert with the European Federation of Academies of Medicine on the deployment of AI in health.

Part I

Drug Innovation for the Benefit of the Patient

High-tech Drugs Against COVID-19

1

Anatomy of a Shared Health Crisis

Five years ago, humanity was faced with a major health crisis. This is now under control, with the end of the global health emergency officially declared on May 5, 2023, by the WHO (World Health Organization). To date, the precise timeline of the start of the COVID-19 pandemic caused by the SARS-CoV-2 coronavirus remains unclear. We know that the virus uses bats as a reservoir animal and that the spread of the virus began in late 2019 at the Wuhan market, in Hubei province in China, before it spread within days across Asia and around the world. In addition to this hypothesis of the transmission of the virus from animal to human, the possibility of the spread of the coronavirus following a containment breach in a Chinese research laboratory is not completely ruled out to this day.

According to WHO figures, by the end of 2024, the SARS-CoV-2 coronavirus had infected more than 775 million people worldwide, causing 7 million officially recorded deaths. However, based on the excess mortality figures observed worldwide in 2020 and 2021, the WHO estimates that the actual number of deaths caused by this pandemic is over 20 million.[1]

The COVID-19 health crisis greatly accelerated the digital transformation of our societies. Thanks to technologies allowing the rapid transmission of information in an ultra-connected world, the global population witnessed in real time the debates shaking the medical and scientific community regarding measures to fight this new virus. Between 2020 and 2021, digital transformation imposed itself in all areas, affecting businesses, administrations, shops, citizens, all countries, and all generations combined. Employees adopted teleworking, patients and doctors used

[1] WHO Coronavirus (COVID-19 Dashboard). By the end of December 2024, COVID-19 had officially caused 7 million deaths worldwide, while more than 13.5 billion doses of vaccine had been administered. According to the WHO, the excess mortality linked to COVID-19 has affected life expectancy in two-thirds of countries.

P. Moingeon, *Intelligent Drugs: How AI is Transforming Healthcare*,
https://doi.org/10.1007/978-3-031-91668-7_1

telemedicine, students and teachers practiced distance learning, consumers and merchants favored online orders, while families exchanged via *Skype* or *FaceTime*. While highlighting how important social interaction is for our well-being, these digital tools have allowed life to continue almost normally.

The COVID-19 pandemic has provided many important lessons. We realized the fragility of our health systems and the lack of hospital infrastructure to cope with the influx of severe cases of COVID-19, requiring heavy and costly care. The damage caused by the virus disrupted global production chains, affecting manufacturing sectors, services, transport, tourism, leisure, entertainment, and culture, even leading to an almost total blockage of the movement of people and goods for many months. The dependence of Western countries on countries like China and India for the production of drugs became evident, thus highlighting the new concern to ensure a "pharmaceutical sovereignty" for these countries. Independence in terms of drugs is now considered strategic at the European level, like aviation, space, armament, or energy. The need to relocate the production of the active ingredients of critical drugs, largely produced in Asia, has become a priority. As an example, the French government announced in June 2023 a reinvestment plan in the industrial production chain to avoid medium-term shortages and allow the relocation of 50 strategic drugs in France.[2]

COVID-19 has also provided lessons on our individual and collective behaviors. We have seen multiple examples of cooperation, remarkable solidarity initiatives, and acts of bravery from healthcare staff and many other professionals who have kept the gears of our societies running. Moreover, we could notice the financial power of developed states that has allowed them to manage the economic consequences of the crisis in the short term, particularly by protecting employment. During the crisis, many countries implemented concerted economic support programs, whereas central banks injected hundreds of billions of euros into the global economy. By mid-2021, the total amount of subsidies implemented or promised by states to support the global economy exceeded USD 10,000 billion!

This crisis has highlighted the importance, but also the complexity, of a global response on a planetary scale to a problem of such magnitude. We have seen some nations helping each other, but also others sometimes guilty of disunity, prioritizing their national interests, or even engaging in geopolitical confrontations through propaganda communication. A COVAX initiative was launched jointly by the WHO and the Global Alliance for Vaccines and Immunization (GAVI), which has financed 1.3 billion doses of vaccines for low-income countries, particularly in Africa. At the same time, we have witnessed vaccine nationalism, denounced at the Davos forum in 2021, by rich countries that have hoarded nearly three-quarters of the vaccine doses produced in the world, mainly for their citizens.

Despite the dramatic aspect of this pandemic in the eyes of the general public, it is far from exceptional for epidemiologists. Humanity has been exposed in history

[2] These strategic drugs include in particular antibiotics, anticancer drugs and anesthetics. As part of this plan, national drug manufacturers are also asked to guarantee at least 4 months of stock for a list of 450 important drugs.

to numerous pathogenic infectious agents responsible for epidemics far deadlier than COVID-19. For example, in the fourteenth century, the Black Death decimated a third of the world's population, or hundreds of millions of people. The Spanish flu caused about 50 million deaths in 1917–1918, and the flu virus caused four large-scale epidemics during the twentieth century. Other coronaviruses distinct from SARS-CoV-2 have also been involved in deadly respiratory diseases, although their impact has been relatively limited during the SARS (*Severe Acute Respiratory Syndrome)* epidemic in 2003 and MERS (*Middle East Respiratory Syndrome*) in 2012.[3]

It is thus important to learn from this COVID-19 pandemic, as it is prototypical of the multiple health problems that threaten humanity and have no borders. In addition to the risk of infectious epidemics, other examples include bacterial resistance to antibiotics as well as diseases related to poverty or environmental degradation. Not implementing appropriate and coordinated measures at the international level to anticipate these risks would make them anthropogenic, as they would then be directly attributable to human irresponsibility. However, the manifest lack of humanity's preparedness for an infectious pandemic risk is one of the main lessons of COVID-19. Bill Gates at a TED conference in 2015, but also the experts gathered by the WHO in 2018 as part of the *Global Preparedness Monitoring Board*, had already warned about the lack of global coordination of authorities in the face of the highly probable risk of a future global infectious epidemic.[4]

In 2022, a commission of scientific experts, coordinated by Professor Jeffrey Sachs, published a detailed report in the journal *The Lancet*, listing the lessons from the COVID-19 crisis to better prepare the response to future comparable situations. This report laments the lack of collaboration and international coordination in handling the transmission of the virus and in implementing effective health measures, such as vaccines, masks, travel regulations, and epidemic tracking tests. The unequal access to care, especially for disadvantaged populations, as well as the lack of cooperation observed in the distribution of vaccines on a global scale, have been particularly identified as points to improve. The commission also criticized the irrational management and disinformation of some governments, notably in China, Brazil,

---

[3] Coronaviruses are a well-known family of RNA viruses, involved in particular in 25% of common winter colds, without severity. The SARS virus, now named SARS-CoV-1, and MERS are however very pathogenic coronaviruses for humans, but which have caused geographically circumscribed epidemics. The mortality rate associated with COVID-19 is estimated at 0.6%, compared to the mortality rate of 3% associated with the Spanish flu pandemic at the beginning of the twentieth century.

[4] See www.ted.com April 3, 2015. Bill Gates [1] and Oppenheim et al. [2]. Also see the website of the World Health Organization https://apps.who.int/gpmb/assets/annual_report/GPMB2019. The *Global Preparedness Monitoring Board* has recommended the creation of independent expert groups to plan for infectious risks that are likely to occur, due to the constant movement of millions of people across the planet. The epidemic risk involving viruses infecting the respiratory tract or causing hemorrhagic fevers is also increased by global warming. Infectious disease experts particularly fear a deadly epidemic linked to highly pathogenic strains of the influenza virus.

and the United States. In this regard, the report particularly recommends educating the population to fight against disinformation and promote prevention approaches.[5]

Some lessons from COVID-19 have been learned. In September 2021, Europe announced the creation of a new agency called HERA (*Health Emergency Response Authority*) to strengthen its ability to prevent, detect, and resolve future health crises. Inspired by the American BARDA, this agency is now in charge of coordinating the development, supply, storage, and distribution of prevention and treatment means to deal with problems similar to COVID-19.[6] In May 2023, the WHO also announced the establishment of a global collaborative network aimed at protecting populations against infectious diseases by performing genomic analyses of large-scale pathogens. These data will eventually be used to make better coordinated public health decisions.

Finally, another major lesson from COVID-19 deserves particular emphasis: the response to this health crisis has revealed the technological power that humanity has today to design and develop new drugs.

When Drug Sciences Meet Artificial Intelligence

COVID-19 has highlighted a remarkable synergy between biotechnologies, nanotechnologies, digital technologies, and AI. Together, these have enabled the ultra-rapid development of effective drugs and vaccines. In less than a year, scientists have managed to develop several innovative vaccines and confirm their effectiveness in humans, an achievement never before accomplished! Traditionally, the development of a new drug takes more than 10 years, as we will see later. These vaccines have proved particularly effective, with protection rates against coronavirus infection exceeding 90% for vaccines used in developed countries and nearly 100% for the prevention of severe forms of the disease, notably respiratory distress.

In addition to the contribution of new technologies, the success of the rapid development of vaccines and treatments against COVID-19 is also explained by the strong commitment to a common cause by different actors driven by the same sense of urgency. Drug manufacturers have taken significant risks by betting on unproven technologies, such as RNA vaccines used by companies like Pfizer or Moderna, or little-used commercial vaccines, like the recombinant adenoviruses developed by AstraZeneca or Johnson & Johnson. In the 1990s, several RNA-based vaccines

[5] Sachs et al. [3]. This commission of experts proposed the creation of a global health fund in collaboration with the WHO, to increase resources to better anticipate emerging diseases and establish rules of international cooperation in the face of such epidemics. The commission also emphasized the need for multilateral collaboration based on United Nations institutions to implement a global plan for managing health emergencies, while protecting individual rights. National and international preparedness plans are recommended to monitor infectious agents, track the use of animal species, enforce biosafety rules in laboratories, and effectively manage stocks of protective equipment, diagnostics, treatments, and vaccines.

[6] *The Biomedical Advanced Research and Development Authority* (BARDA) is the agency created in the United States to fight against pandemics, emerging diseases, and bioterrorism.

were tested in humans to fight against cancers or viral infections. These developments have encountered the instability of RNA molecules, which rapidly degrade after administration in the body. In the case of vaccines against SARS-CoV-2, this problem was solved by using nanolipidic formulations to protect the RNAs.

These achievements were made possible thanks to a close collaboration between academic and industrial researchers and between biotechs and pharmaceutical giants, with the support of policymakers. In addition to the investments of billions of euros by industry, many states and philanthropic organizations have made a substantial financial contribution. These contributions have accelerated the development of drugs and vaccines against COVID-19, notably thanks to initiatives such as *Warp Speed* in the United States, as well as the CEPI alliance (*Coalition for Epidemic Preparedness Innovations*) on a global scale. This alliance has brought together vaccine developers and manufacturers, about 30 states, the *Bill and Melinda Gates Foundation,* and the *Wellcome Trust* to finance the production of Moderna, AstraZeneca, and Novavax's anti-COVID-19 vaccines. This crisis has illustrated the importance, but also the complexity, of a global response on a planetary scale to a problem of such magnitude.

Regulatory agencies also deserve special mention, as they have played an important role in managing the health emergency by adapting the usual rules for drug evaluation. In practice, the review of vaccine registration files and their approval by the American (*Food and Drug Administration*, FDA) and European (*European Medicines Agency*, EMA) health authorities took less than a month, instead of 1–2 years outside emergency situations (see Box 1.1).

Box 1.1: An Unprecedented Regulatory Evaluation of Anti-COVID-19 Vaccines

The management of the emergency of the health crisis related to COVID-19 constitutes a case study on the regulatory level. Health agencies worked closely with the industry for the design and implementation of clinical studies evaluating the effectiveness and safety of vaccines. In particular, these studies were conducted in parallel rather than sequentially, and their results were analyzed extremely quickly. The large-scale production processes for candidate vaccines were developed in anticipation, even before knowing if they were effective. The majority of vaccines were thus quickly tested in clinical studies involving 30,000–40,000 healthy adults who volunteered.

Following the positive results of these studies, the FDA and EMA gave their green light for a temporary authorization for the use of vaccines against COVID-19. This marketing authorization was accompanied by an obligation for manufacturers to conduct specific clinical studies in children, the very elderly, or those with particular comorbidities, notably diseases of the immune system. As the vaccines were deployed on a large scale to millions, then billions of people, all adverse effects were collected and analyzed to confirm, *in fine,* their satisfactory safety profile.

The COVID-19 pandemic has confirmed the remarkable effectiveness of vaccines in the fight against infectious diseases. In the case of SARS-CoV-2, the vaccines aimed to stimulate in humans an immune response to a virus protein called *Spike*. This was chosen for two essential reasons: it is expressed on the surface of the virus and is necessary for it to infect human cells. After the administration of the RNA vaccines, only the protein *Spike* is expressed in the body in the absence of infectious viral particles. The immune system of the vaccinated individual then produces anti-*Spike* antibodies capable of neutralizing the virus in the event of subsequent natural exposure. The results demonstrating the effectiveness of vaccines on very large cohorts of subjects have been published in prestigious scientific journals, such as the *New England Journal of Medicine* [4, 5]. This effectiveness has also been widely confirmed after their market release on a population scale. From the beginning of 2021, countries such as the United Kingdom, Israel, and the United States, where a significant proportion (50–60%) of the population had received at least one dose of these vaccines, have seen a significant decrease in infection and mortality rates. It is estimated that, thanks to vaccines, 20 million deaths have already been prevented in the first year of their deployment.[7]

In addition to these preventive vaccines for infection and disease, various drugs developed and tested in humans during 2020 and 2021 have been made available to treat COVID-19. These drugs, presented below in Table 1.1, include various monoclonal anti-*Spike* antibodies that neutralize the virus, as well as synthetic chemical molecule-based antivirals that block its replication. They are useful for combating SARS-CoV-2 in patients infected by mechanisms complementary to those of vaccines, preventing the progression to severe forms of the disease.

The development of vaccines and effective treatments in 1 year is an achievement made possible thanks to not only bio- and nanotechnologies but also digital technologies and AI. Biotechnologies have enabled the development of vaccines based on RNA and on proteins or recombinant viruses; nanotechnologies have provided the formulations to prevent the degradation of RNAs after administration. Biotechnologies have also been used to produce industrial-scale quantities of vaccines. The availability in 3 years of 13.5 billion doses of vaccines distributed worldwide is an unprecedented performance in large-scale drug production and distribution!

AI has played a crucial role in integrating and analyzing large amounts of data collected on the virus and its evolution, thanks to digital technologies. It has been used to interpret the genomic sequences of the coronavirus obtained from the millions of samples taken worldwide, thus allowing the detection of emerging new variants. These analyses have led to the creation of computer models to track in real time the spread of the SARS-CoV-2 virus and guide the fight against the pandemic

[7] Watson et al. [6]. At the same time, countries lagging in the deployment of these vaccines, including notably many European countries, have been faced with a resurgence of infections, hospitalizations, and mortality, forcing them to confine their populations for the third time. In these lagging countries, healthcare systems have been severely challenged by the explosion of severe forms of the disease.

Table 1.1 Available drugs against COVID-19

Drugs (laboratories)	Characteristics
Preventive vaccines RNA formulated as lipid nanoparticles: Spikevax® (Moderna), Comirnaty® (Pfizer/BNTX) Adeno-associated virus expressing the *Spike* protein: Vaxzevria® (AstraZeneca/University of Oxford), Jcovden® (Johnson & Johnson) Subunit vaccine (recombinant *Spike* protein): Nuvaxovid® (Novavax), VidPrevtyn Beta® (Sanofi/GSK) Whole inactivated virus-based vaccine: VLA200® (Valneva)	All vaccines (except VLA2001) are based on the *Spike* protein expressed on the surface of the SARS-CoV-2 virus and are presented in different forms. These vaccines generally require two injections (with the exception of the one from Johnson & Johnson, which requires only one administration). They protect very effectively against severe forms of the disease, thus preventing hospitalization in intensive care. The VLA200® vaccine from Valneva, based on a whole inactivated virus, is authorized for primary vaccination in adults In 2021, several variants of the virus (Alpha, Beta, Delta, and Omicron) appeared after mutations of the original Wuhan strain, which could potentially question the effectiveness of vaccines and drugs already developed. To date, the immunity induced by vaccines has proven effective against all major variants observed, to varying degrees. Protective immunity, especially antibodies neutralizing the virus, tends to decrease after 6 months. A booster vaccination (third dose) was implemented in most countries at the end of 2021, with a fourth dose recommended for those over 60 years old. Second- and third-generation vaccines were then developed to better protect against Omicron subvariants that appeared in 2022 The side effects of these vaccines are limited, most often minor (fever, fatigue, pain at the injection site, muscle or joint pain, flu-like symptoms). A few rare cases of severe allergic or anaphylactic reactions, myocarditis, pericarditis, and thrombosis have been reported. The benefit–risk ratio of these vaccines remains very positive[a]
Neutralizing monoclonal antibodies Ronapreve® (Roche/Regeneron) Bamlanivimab®/Etesevimab® (Eli Lilly) Xevudy® (GSK) Evusheld® (AstraZeneca)	These antibodies directed against the *Spike* protein allow for the rapid neutralization of the virus. They are used to treat patients already infected and prevent the progression to severe forms of COVID-19, characterized by strong inflammation in the lungs. The effectiveness of these monoclonal antibodies varies depending on the variants involved. Several of them have proven effective against the Omicron variant, as well as its subvariants observed in 2022
Antivirals (small synthetic chemical molecules) Remdesivir® (Gilead) Molnupiravir® (Merck) Paxlovid® (Pfizer)	Oral antivirals have been developed to treat patients with mild or moderate COVID-19, whenever at risk of developing severe forms due to concomitant pathologies (obesity, hypertension, diabetes, cardiovascular diseases, and immunosuppression) These drugs are directed against different enzymes involved in the metabolism of the virus (RNA polymerase or protease), thus preventing its replication

(continued)

Table 1.1 (continued)

Drugs (laboratories)	Characteristics
Repositioned anti-inflammatory drugs	Several existing anti-inflammatory drugs have been repositioned in the treatment of COVID-19, such as dexamethasone, interleukin 6 antagonists (Tocilizumab®), or JAK family kinase inhibitors (Tofacitinib®, Baricitinib®). These drugs have been administered to patients who are likely to progress to an acute respiratory syndrome following the hyperactivation of immune cells responsible for a cytokine storm

[a]COVID-19: *Suivi des cas d'effets indésirables des vaccins,* June 2022. Ansm.sante.fr. The Russian (Sputnik V) and Chinese (Sinovac, Sinopharm) vaccines have—in light of the results of phase 2 clinical studies published in scientific journals—shown lower efficacy than those developed by Western countries. Their efficacy also appears to be reduced against new variants of the virus, notably Omicron. These vaccines are not authorized by the regulatory agencies of the European Union, nor of North America. However, they have been approved by the WHO to allow vaccination of adults in developing countries

by coordinating barrier measures and care at the national and international level. At the molecular level, AI has also allowed us to model the interactions between the virus and the infected human cells. These models have accurately revealed the effective immune defense mechanisms against the virus as well as their dysfunction in patients with severe forms of COVID-19. Other models have been created to predict possible variations in its *Spike* protein, which allows the SARS-CoV-2 virus to escape the immune system while remaining capable of infecting human cells. Simulations of the disease's evolution toward severe pulmonary inflammatory forms have also been carried out, opening the way to new therapeutic targets. AI has also been used to predict, from medical records, which patients were likely to develop long COVID or to manifest rare side effects after vaccination, such as myocarditis.

Collectively, all this knowledge generated quickly, thanks to AI, has proven extremely valuable in helping the health industry to develop innovative vaccines, predict the response of different virus variants to drugs, and reposition existing drugs to treat COVID-19 (Table 1.1). The fight against COVID-19 has also confirmed the power of biotechnologies, demonstrating the interest and flexibility of RNA technology to produce vaccines against pathogens capable of great genetic variability. Humanity has been able to quickly win the battle against the SARS-CoV-2 virus and its variants thanks to the encounter between AI and biotechnology. According to experts, COVID-19 will be managed in the future like recurrent episodes of the flu, with regular booster vaccinations against new forms of the virus, with the aim of preventing severe infections.

Who to Believe, Between Scientific Experts and Social Networks?

Despite the successes in the fight against COVID-19, everyone has been able to observe, unexpectedly, a growing distrust in public opinion toward health measures and vaccines. In many Western countries, demonstrations have taken place against confinement measures, mask wearing, vaccination, and health passes. These movements have reflected the loss of confidence in institutions, especially in Southern Europe (France, Spain, and Italy) and North America. This low credibility of governments seems partly linked to the perceived inequalities in protection against this anxiety-inducing health crisis.[8]

In such a context, public opinion could easily be manipulated by false information exchanged on social networks. A mix of unsupported opinions, pseudo-scientific beliefs, and coffee shop opinions often made real scientific expertise inaudible. As a result, a portion of the population rejected the COVID-19 vaccines, despite factual evidence of their effectiveness and safety. Detractors of the anti-COVID-19 vaccines questioned the available information on these vaccines and spread implausible conspiracy theories about the origin of the pandemic while expressing a pronounced distrust not only of the governments but also of the pharmaceutical industry and scientific experts. While the introduction in many countries of a health pass linked to vaccination aimed to regain the freedom to safely frequent public places, this measure was accused of restricting individual freedoms. The heightened mistrust among a fraction of the population toward anti-COVID-19 vaccines had the tragic consequence that unvaccinated people developed severe forms—or even died—from COVID-19 out of ignorance, even though effective vaccines were available. One controversy in particular concerned the side effects related to vaccines. Although well tolerated by the vast majority of vaccinated individuals, a few infrequent adverse effects have been reported, some considered serious, such as anaphylactic reactions, myocarditis, or thrombosis (Table 1.1). In France, these serious adverse effects affected 2.5 people out of 10,000 vaccinated, mainly in populations with well-identified susceptibilities, for whom medical observation after vaccination minimized the risk. As we will see later, this is a classic situation in which otherwise very effective drugs can cause, apart from minor and temporary local reactions, objective but infrequent adverse effects. In 2024, with the hindsight of several years of use on a population scale, the confirmation of a very favorable benefit-to-risk ratio fully justifies the use of these anti-COVID-19 vaccines, particularly to avoid severe, even fatal, forms of the disease.

Ironically, some unfounded treatments were ardently defended, often by the same vaccine skeptics! A notable example in Europe concerns hydroxychloroquine, a drug used to treat malaria and certain autoimmune diseases, which was proposed to fight against COVID-19. This hypothesis, actively promoted in France by Didier Raoult in the context of the prevailing emergency at the beginning of the pandemic,

[8] Eurofound e-survey 2020. *Living, working and COVID-19 dataset Dublin*: http://eurofound.link/covid19data

was then documented on a very small number of patients, with a questionable methodology regarding the control group used. The effectiveness of hydroxychloroquine was therefore the subject of two large-scale clinical studies, meeting the methodological quality requirements to be used in the evaluation of a drug in humans. These studies, unfortunately, demonstrated with certainty, as early as 2020, a total lack of effectiveness of hydroxychloroquine in COVID-19, with, moreover, severe hepatic and cardiac side effects observed in some patients [7, 8].

The success of the development of vaccines and anti-COVID-19 drugs highlighted the societal utility of the pharmaceutical industry. European public opinion has often been quick to criticize an industry "making profits from the health problems of the population." When asked about this, Albert Bourla, the CEO of Pfizer, a major commercial winner from the success of the anti-COVID-19 vaccines, emphasized that his company had taken considerable financial risks to develop and produce these vaccines. He also recalled the great societal value of these drugs, which have prevented the hospitalization and death of many patients and, beyond that, avoided a cataclysmic disruption of global economic activities. A reassuring opinion survey, conducted in France by the IPSOS institute for LEEM (the professional organization of drug companies), confirmed an improvement in the image of pharmaceutical companies among the general public, health professionals, and officials by the end of 2021.[9]

The mistrust observed toward vaccines highlights the need to fight against irrationality linked to ignorance. The debates and controversies over anti-COVID-19 vaccines foreshadow those to come on future drugs, opposing societal interest and individual freedom, but also expert knowledge and public opinion, the latter being subject to various manipulations. Vaccination has the particularity of aiming to prevent disease in healthy individuals. However, as we will see later, in the coming decades, a major evolution supported by AI will be the emergence of drugs aimed at preventing diseases, not just curing them. The mistrust toward anti-COVID-19 vaccines is therefore a foretaste of the ambivalence that a part of the population will be tempted to show toward intelligent drugs intended to avoid diseases not yet declared.

[9] This survey reflects an improvement in confidence towards the pharmaceutical industry, but also towards drugs and vaccines. More than 90% of the French acknowledged at the end of 2021 the usefulness of the pharmaceutical industry. The public gives it 62% of its trust, whereas only 52% did so in 2019. The residual criticisms focus on the profits made by the health industry, the lack of transparency during the fight against COVID-19, as well as the absence of French-origin vaccines against COVID-19. On this last point, the VLA2001® vaccine from the Franco-Austrian company Valvena received its market authorization in Europe in June 2022.

References

1. Bill Gates. The next outbreak? We're not ready. April 3rd 2015. https://www.ted.com
2. Oppenheim B, et al. The world needs an intergovernmental panel on pandemic risk. Nat Med. 2021;27:934.
3. Sachs J et al. The Lancet Commission on lessons for the future from the COVID-19 pandemic. www.thelancet.com. 14 Sept 2022.
4. Polack F, et al. Safety and efficacy of the BNT162b2 mRNA Covid-19 vaccine. New Engl J Med. 2020;383:2603.
5. Baden L, et al. Efficacy and safety of the mRNA-1273 SARS-CoV-2 vaccine. New Engl J Med. 2021;384:403.
6. Watson O, et al. Global impact of the first year of Covid 19 vaccination: a mathematical modelling study. Lancet Infect Dis. 2022;9:1293.
7. Boulware D, et al. A randomized trial of hydroxychloroquine as postexposure prophylaxis for Covid-19. New Engl J Med. 2020;383:517.
8. The RECOVERY Collaborative Group. Effect of hydroxychloroquine in hospitalized patients with Covid-19. New Engl J Med. 2020;383:2030.

Behind the Scenes of an Exponential Innovation

2

From the First Drugs to Biological Medicines

The history of drugs, closely linked to that of medicine, is based on a constant evolution of practices, knowledge, and technologies in two areas of expertise, respectively carried out by apothecaries and the first doctors.[1] Over time, observation gave way to experimentation and then to scientific conceptualization, promoting the cross-fertilization and enrichment of knowledge. Schematically, this history is structured around three periods. A magical-empirical approach initially, used in ancient times to discover the first drugs, gave way to the gradual development of modern drugs as we know them, followed by the very recent emergence of intelligent drugs resulting from accelerated innovation, which interests us here.

From Antiquity to the Middle Ages, drugs were obtained from substances present in nature. The first known drug collections, called pharmacopoeias, are the Sumerian tablets of Nipur and the Chinese *Shennong bencao jing*, both dating from about 2900 years before our era, to which was added the Egyptian pharmacopoeia recorded in the Ebers papyrus (1600 BC). These documents list the first drugs discovered by humanity in the form of extracts or concoctions of plants, minerals, or animal tissues.[2] The first apothecaries continued to list natural products with

[1]The history of drug sciences has been the subject of numerous dedicated works to which the reader can refer for more details. Among these: O. Lafont, *Apothicaires et pharmaciens. Histoire d'une conquête scientifique*, John Libbey, 2021; F. Chast, *Histoire contemporaine du medicament*. La Découverte, 1995; É. Perrot, *La connaissance des drogues simples d'origine végétale.* Maretheux and Pactat, 1932.

[2]These first pharmacopoeias mention, for example, plants with sedative virtues (poppy, henbane), purgatives (senna, castor oil, colocynth), diuretic (squill), as well as opium and the mandrake. Minerals such as ochre, or blood, bones and animal fats are also mentioned to treat human afflictions.

P. Moingeon, *Intelligent Drugs: How AI is Transforming Healthcare*,
https://doi.org/10.1007/978-3-031-91668-7_2

therapeutic virtues without understanding their mechanisms of action. At the same time, medicine was born in the ancient Greco-Roman world with Hippocrates (fifth century BC) and progressed thanks to scholars like Galen (second century AD) and Avicenna (eleventh century AD). An emblematic drug designed at this time is the famous Theriac, a mixture of about 50 drugs, plants, and minerals, used as a treatment against poisonings and bites of venomous animals.[3] Pliny the Elder (first century AD), apparently not convinced of its effectiveness, then qualified this Theriac as "vain ostentation of science and monstrous charlatanism"!

However, over time, advances in knowledge have allowed the emergence of first principles to explain "medical realities." At the end of the first millennium, a major event took place: the encounter between the knowledge hitherto separated from the apothecaries, experts in drugs, and the doctors, concerned to understand diseases. This period also saw the first attempts to isolate active substances from natural sources. Latin texts, including the *Antidotarium Nicolai* and successive versions of the *De Materia Medica,* established increasingly precise rules for the use of these drugs in the Middle Ages, listing their effects on human or animal diseases.

In the sixteenth century, Paracelsus, both a doctor and an alchemist, embodied the transition to the modern period based on science. This scholar is the first to explicitly advocate the use of specific drugs to treat a given disease. Progress accelerated in the eighteenth and nineteenth centuries in multiple disciplines, such as chemistry with Antoine Lavoisier, physiology and experimental medicine with Claude Bernard, pharmacology with Rudolf Buchheim, and vaccination with Edward Jenner and Louis Pasteur. Scientists then tried to understand, reproduce, and manipulate in the laboratory the multiple medicinal potentialities identified in nature. The medical approach evolved from observation to experimentation with Claude Bernard, allowing a better understanding of the functioning of the human body by establishing links between causes and effects. The therapeutic approach was progressively structured around scientific concepts nourished by iterations between theories, hypotheses, and experiments.

In the nineteenth century, advances in chemistry made it possible to isolate and characterize many active principles from plants, such as morphine, codeine, quinine, emetine, and ergotamine. But also, at the end of this century, to produce them in the laboratory, thus marking the birth of the pharmaceutical industry. Acetylsalicylic acid, the active principle of aspirin, was synthesized by Felix Hoffman in 1897, followed at the beginning of the twentieth century by the chemical synthesis of the first local anesthetics, antisyphilitics, and antimalarials. The period that followed saw the gradual emergence of different classes of drugs as we know them today. More natural molecules of therapeutic interest were produced in the laboratory, and it became possible to modify them to improve their effectiveness as well as their stability in the

[3] Conceived in the ancient world and perfected by the Cretan physician Andromachus (first century AD), then by Galen, the Theriac contained among other things opium, castoreum, squill and viper flesh... Its composition continued to enrich with the knowledge and imagination of apothecaries until the seventeenth century.

body while reducing their undesirable effects. The pharmacopoeia was considerably enriched from the middle of the twentieth century, with many new drug molecules that were effective and better tolerated. At the same time, the rules for using a drug to treat a disease, the dosage, and contraindications were gradually established on the basis of scientific reasoning. A rigorous methodology was also defined for clinical studies evaluating in humans the effectiveness and safety of new treatments within the framework of a medicine now based on evidence.[4]

At the beginning of the 1980s, a new engine of drug innovation appeared, driven by biotechnologies resulting from advances in cellular, molecular, and genetic biology. The resolution of the structure of DNA and the genetic code in the 1950s, the understanding of gene regulation mechanisms at the end of the twentieth century, and the sequencing of the human genome at the beginning of the third millennium offered new insights into vital biological processes and their deregulation in diseases. Medicine quickly integrated this molecular knowledge into its diagnostics and treatments, complementing the clinical description of symptoms with biological data and medical imaging to represent diseases with more precision.

Biotechnologies are defined as the application of science and technology to living organisms to produce knowledge, goods, or services. Concretely, these technologies allow the manipulation of living organisms by transferring genes from one organism to another. With the new possibility of inserting into bacteria, yeasts, insect or human cells, plants or animals, diverse genes coding for therapeutic proteins of interest, biotechnologies have allowed the emergence within 20 years of a new class of biological drugs.[5] These include human therapeutic proteins (insulin, growth hormones, coagulation factors, and cytokines), monoclonal antibodies, vaccines, natural products derived from human blood, as well as cell or gene therapy products. Collectively, they now represent more than half of the new drugs developed by the pharmaceutical industry.

As a result, at the end of the twentieth century, two major categories of modern drugs were available in pharmacies, depending on whether they were produced by chemical synthesis or derived from biotechnology.[6] These two families of drugs contributed to shaping contemporary medicine.

---

[4] Numerous major drug classes have been developed during the twentieth century by a pharmaceutical industry based on synthetic chemistry. Let's mention here a few important milestones, with their discovery dates: Antihistamines (1942), Coumarin anticoagulants (1947), Hypoglycemic sulfonamides (1949). As for antibiotics: discovery of Penicillin by Fleming (1928), Tetracyclines (1948), Ampicillin (1961), Amoxicillin (1964). Antitubercular: discovery of Streptomycin (1946) and Isoniazid (1952). Anti-inflammatories: Cortisone (1949). Regarding psychotropics: neuroleptics (1950), monoamine oxidase inhibitors and imipraminic antidepressants (1957). Contraceptives: development by Pincus of the first pill based on Progesterone (1960). Betablockers: Propranolol (1967). First antiviral inhibitors of the AIDS virus: Zidovudine® (1985).

[5] These host cells, genetically modified, produce the protein coded by the transfected gene. The proteins thus produced by a cell whose genetic material has been modified by genetic recombination are called recombinant proteins.

[6] Drugs can also be classified according to their pharmacological properties or their use in the treatment of specific organ diseases. See www.leem.org/ *Comment classe-t-on les médicaments*; www.wikipedia.org/ *Catégories de médicaments*.

Fifty Years of the Success of Modern Drugs

Chemical drugs have, in recent years, achieved major victories against deadly viral diseases associated with HIV (Human Immunodeficiency Virus, responsible for AIDS) and the hepatitis C virus. Thanks to antiretroviral drugs developed in the late 1980s to combat HIV, the life expectancy of infected people is now similar to that of the general population, whereas at the beginning of the epidemic, these patients were condemned in the short term, except for exceptional cases, nicknamed *long-term survivors*. Although the virus is not yet eradicated, with still 38 million HIV-positive people in the world, the epidemic is receding, and some experts even envisage a possible eradication of AIDS by 2030 by treating recently infected subjects to prevent the transmission of the virus, but also preventively, those at high risk of exposure to the virus.[7]

In the 1970s, the hepatitis C virus, which is responsible for severe liver diseases, was discovered. This virus causes chronic infections leading to persistent inflammation of the liver, which can progress to cirrhosis and even cancer. In 2014, the development of the drug Solvadi® by Gilead Sciences revolutionized the treatment of hepatitis C, allowing 95% of patients to be cured after only a few weeks of treatment! Solvadi has attracted a lot of attention, not only because of its remarkable effectiveness in a disease hitherto poorly treated but also because of its high price, thus raising the question of the cost of new innovative treatments, on which we will return.[8]

On the other hand, several classes of chemical drugs have also made spectacular progress in the management of many cardiovascular diseases. Thiazide diuretic-based antihypertensives, angiotensin receptor antagonists, calcium inhibitors, and beta-blockers have significantly improved the treatment of high blood pressure. Antiarrhythmic drugs are used to prevent and treat heart rhythm disorders. In stroke, a tissue plasminogen activator is used to dissolve blood clots that block blood vessels, whereas anticoagulants and platelet antiaggregants are used to prevent their formation. Hypolipidemic statins have been developed to lower blood cholesterol levels, thus preventing the development and worsening of atherosclerosis, reducing the incidence of coronary artery disease, and ultimately lowering the risk of myocardial infarction. To fully understand the impact of all these therapeutic advances,

[7] In the early 1980s, mankind discovered the human immunodeficiency virus or HIV, previously unknown, capable of destroying CD4+ T lymphocytes, central cells in the functioning of the immune system. Researchers quickly developed increasingly effective antiretroviral drugs, then learned to combine these molecules to prevent the resistance of the virus to treatment. Today, it is estimated that more than 60% of HIV-positive patients worldwide receive these drugs, which allows them to no longer transmit the virus. A current aim is to preventively treat people at high risk of exposure to the virus, as part of what is called a pre-exposure prophylactic antiviral treatment.

[8] For the hepatitis C virus as for the HIV virus, attempts to develop a vaccine have so far been unsuccessful due to the very high genetic variability of these two viruses, capable of evolving through mutations into numerous subtypes that escape the immune system.

it should be remembered that nearly 40% of the 60 million annual deaths worldwide are related to these cardiovascular diseases.[9]

Another very recent innovation constitutes a revolution in the management of overweight patients. Analogues of the hormone GLP1 in the form of synthetic peptides initially used in the treatment of type 2 diabetes in overweight patients are now offered to obese people. In this latter indication, the results are comparable to those of the surgical approaches, allowing the weight of the treated patients to be reduced by 20–25%. We will return later to this new class of drugs that has the ability to reduce the incidence of more than 200 pathologies associated with obesity. Among these, the risk of cardiovascular diseases, such as heart failure, hypertension, and strokes, as well as cancers associated with obesity. This new therapeutic class could thus improve the quality of life of many patients and contribute to extending the duration of a healthy life.

In parallel, biotechnologies have greatly enriched the pharmacopoeia by allowing the large-scale production of multiple human proteins of therapeutic interest. For example, human insulin produced by genetic engineering in the early 1980s replaced pig insulin, which was previously extracted from animal tissues, to treat patients with diabetes. Similarly, interferon α2a in 1980 and erythropoietin in 1988 were produced in the laboratory to stimulate the immune system and the production of red blood cells, respectively. Biotechnologies have also made it possible to more precisely target abnormal cells or tissues thanks to monoclonal antibodies, nicknamed "magic bullets" because of their great specificity for a molecular target. These monoclonal antibodies have revolutionized the treatment of various pathologies, such as cancers or age-related retinal degeneration, in light of their remarkable ability to recognize targets of interest. Biotherapies based on antibodies that very selectively inhibit cytokines activating the immune system, such as TNFα or interleukin 1, have thus transformed the lives of millions of patients suffering from inflammatory diseases, such as rheumatoid arthritis or Crohn's disease.[10]

Biotechnologies have also given a new impetus to vaccines. Historically, these were produced from infectious agents—viruses or bacteria—inactivated or attenuated by heat or chemical treatment.[11] Thanks to biotechnologies, molecular vaccines

[9] In comparison, cancer mortality only accounts for a quarter of deaths worldwide. However, in wealthy countries, the incidence of cardiovascular diseases has decreased following better prevention and better treatments, and it is now cancers that cause the most victims. Globally, cardiovascular diseases, however, remain the leading cause of mortality among middle-aged adults, especially in developing countries, where they remain exposed to a risk of dying from a heart disease 2.5 times higher than in wealthy countries.

[10] See Dzau et al. [1]. Monoclonal antibodies also have numerous applications in diagnosis, particularly in the detection or dosage of molecules of interest in biological fluids.

[11] These modified microbes are no longer pathogenic, but they can still induce strong immune responses, which will protect the vaccinated person in case of natural exposure to the infectious agent. This is how many vaccines commonly used against viral diseases such as polio, measles, rubella, mumps or the flu have been produced—and are still manufactured.

based on proteins and/or carbohydrates purified from pathogens have been developed. These vaccines are, for example, used to prevent viral diseases such as hepatitis B, meningitis B, infections with oncogenic papillomaviruses, or pneumococci. More recently, we discussed the contribution of biotechnologies to the development of RNA vaccines against COVID-19.

For more than four decades, these life technologies have allowed the health industry to maintain an extremely rich drug pipeline. The field of oncology has been the main beneficiary of this revolution, with a very large number of biological drugs made available to patients. These new drugs, mostly based on monoclonal antibodies, stand out for their remarkable effectiveness, linked to an ultra-specific targeting of a molecular characteristic specific to the tumor, absent from normal cells. Up to 80% of newly approved treatments in oncology belong to this category. In association with immunotherapies that stimulate natural immune defenses against cancer cells, these drugs have contributed to a spectacular reduction in mortality due to cancers in developed countries.[12]

Most cancers are indeed now considered chronic diseases, thanks to these new treatments that allow people to live longer with the disease, even if the lifespan varies depending on the type of cancer. Overall, the average 10-year survival rate for patients after a cancer diagnosis is now 50%, the same rate observed 1 year after diagnosis in the 1980s! In the United States, lung cancer-related mortality has decreased by 43% in men and 17% in women over the past 15 years, while colorectal cancer mortality has decreased by over 50% for all patients. Death rates from leukemia have also decreased by over 30% in the last 10 years. At the same time, the 10-year survival rates for breast cancer and prostate cancer have significantly increased, rising from 40% to 78% and from 25% to 84%, respectively. These medical advances, achieved in part with newly available drugs from biotechnology, have saved millions of human lives.

A single figure alone summarizes the considerable benefits brought in recent years by modern medicines, namely the increase in human life expectancy. This has almost doubled in the twentieth century thanks to new treatments, vaccination, and advances in hygiene. According to the WHO, since the beginning of the twenty-first century, life expectancy has increased by 5 years. In most developed countries, it is now around 80 years. However, it should be noted that the recent COVID-19 pandemic has led to an average decrease of 1.6 years in life expectancy worldwide. In

[12] Among these targeted biological drugs, there are in particular two monoclonal antibodies directed against the PD 1 protein expressed by certain cells of the immune system. Opdivo® (from Bristol Myers Squibb) has proven very effective in the treatment of head and neck cancer, a disease that affects 600,000 people worldwide each year. Along with Merck's Keytruda®, these two immunotherapy drugs have improved the treatment of melanomas, as well as lung and kidney cancers. They work by lifting the inhibition of the immune system caused by many tumors. With a similar mechanism of action, the anti-CTLA-4 monoclonal antibody Yervoy® (from Bristol Myers Squibb) has also improved the treatment of 20% of patients with metastatic melanoma. These immune checkpoint inhibitors are now being tested in many clinical studies, alone or in combination with other anticancer therapies, for example chemotherapies. The decrease in cancer mortality has also benefited from the reduction in tobacco consumption, as well as the earlier diagnosis of the disease.

France, in 2022, life expectancy was estimated at 79.3 years for men and 85.2 years for women, according to the National Institute of Demographic Studies.[13]

Intelligent Drugs and Precision Medicine

Before outlining what is meant by "intelligent" drugs, let's recall the general characteristics of a drug. The definition common to all countries of the European Union encompasses under this term "*any substance or composition presented as having curative or preventive properties with regard to human or animal diseases, as well as any substance or composition that can be used in humans or animals or can be administered to them, with the aim of obtaining a medical diagnosis or restoring, correcting or modifying their physiological functions by exerting a pharmacological, immunological or metabolic action.*"

The heart of the drug is the active ingredient, that is, the chemical or biological molecule that acts on a dysregulated molecular process in a disease to stimulate it or inhibit it, as the case may be. The mode of action of the active ingredient (pharmacological, immunological, or metabolic) refers to the nature of the modified process. The active ingredient is not administered alone; it is associated with excipients, such as preservatives, diluents, and coating agents, which do not have a medicinal activity. Their role is rather to stabilize the active ingredient and facilitate its galenic formulation, that is, the presentation of the drug in the form of a tablet, capsule, suppository, syrup, solution, injectable solution, skin patch, or inhalable aerosol. Before being made available to patients in pharmacies, the drug must obtain a marketing authorization from public regulatory agencies, according to modalities that we will discuss later.[14]

A drug can be identified under different names. For example, aspirin is known under the international common denomination of its active ingredient (acetylsalicylic acid) but also under various brand names (Alka-Seltzer®, Aspro®, and Aspegic®), which vary according to the pharmaceutical laboratories.[15]

---

[13] According to Wikipedia, life expectancy at birth is the average lifespan of a hypothetical population that would live its entire existence under the mortality conditions of the year considered. There remain significant disparities between countries in life expectancy, which remains for example below 60 years in sub-Saharan Africa. On an individual scale, lifestyle plays an important role. According to the European study *Lifepath*, smoking is associated with a loss of life expectancy of 4.8 years, diabetes of 3.9 years and sedentary lifestyle of 2.4 years. Living in unfavorable socioeconomic conditions would result in a loss of 2 years of life. This life expectancy has been declining since 2015 in the USA, partly explained by addictions to opioids linked to the inappropriate use of painkillers. Due to great inequality in access to care, COVID-19 has also reduced the life expectancy of Americans by an average of 2.7 years.

[14] Some drugs are only available in a hospital setting, when they can only be prescribed by specialists or when they are used to treat rare diseases. Drugs that have received temporary authorization for use are also exclusively dispensed by the hospital, as long as they are still under development.

[15] The real name of the drug is the international nonproprietary name, used since 2015 by doctors in their prescriptions. The R surrounded by a circle on drug boxes, ®, indicates that it is a registered trademark.

From these considerations, how can AI make drugs "intelligent"? In this essay, we will thus qualify any drug designed on a strong scientific rationale, ultra-targeted against a very specific biological process, and intended for patients with well-defined characteristics. We will see that the creation of such drugs is now possible thanks to a convergence of technologies to both obtain data on the patient, analyze these data in order to create predictive models (this is a major contribution of AI), and finally use these models to design treatments adapted according to the characteristics of the patients.

Regarding the perfectly targeted biological mechanism of action of these new drugs, it is based on the specific recognition by the active ingredient of a target altered in the patient, guaranteeing not only its effectiveness but also its safety by avoiding an unwanted interaction with other targets. This property is the consequence of an optimal complementarity at the molecular level between the spatial structure of the active ingredient and that of its target, at the heart of the mechanism of action. For the anecdote, the concept of specific interaction based on the complementarity of shapes between the drug molecule and the therapeutic target is inspired by the work carried out 120 years ago by the German biologist Paul Ehrlich, by analogy with a key opening a lock.[16]

Today, with the availability of various forms of AI, it is possible to model with a computer this molecular interaction at the Angstrom scale (10^{-10} m). For example, the AlphaFold algorithm, recently developed by the company DeepMind, can be used to predict the three-dimensional structure of the majority of proteinaceous targets. With this information, equipped with Oculus-type virtual reality headsets, researchers can "walk around" a giant three-dimensional image of the active principle-target complex to optimize the chemical structure of the drug so that it fits perfectly into the target.[17]

The precise targeting of the smart drug also comes from the fact that it is directed against the appropriate therapeutic target for the considered patient. Consequently, the development of drugs with such a property requires a detailed knowledge of the disease and the diversity of patients, at the basis of what is called precision medicine. This is a major paradigm shift, as, unlike the traditional approach where all patients with a disease receive the same drug, precision medicine now aims to offer a more personalized treatment, which takes into account the characteristics of each individual.[18]

---

[16] Strebhardt and Ullrich [2]. Paul Ehrlich was interested in the interactions between antigens and antibodies, work for which he received the Nobel Prize in Medicine in 1908.

[17] To study the spatial interaction between the active principle of the drug and its target, researchers use physical structural analysis techniques, such as X-ray diffraction, nuclear magnetic resonance or electron cryomicroscopy. These methods are now complemented by the prediction using the AlphaFold algorithm of the three-dimensional structure of proteinaceous therapeutic targets from their amino acid sequence, easily determined by mass spectrometry.

[18] Medicine is thus evolving towards more customized treatments based on the characteristics of patients, instead of a "one size fits all" type approach.

Precision medicine emerged about 15 years ago, when the first cancer treatments targeting specific tumor mutations demonstrated remarkable efficacy in some patients. As an example, Trastuzumab®, a drug based on a monoclonal antibody, proved very effective in 30% of patients with breast cancer expressing the HER2 marker, as confirmed by a diagnostic test. Several other drugs restricted to patients with genetic specificity have allowed, in recent years, for improved effectiveness of treatments against various cancers while reducing their toxicity.[19] Following these successes, the FDA approved in 2017 the marketing of Keytruda®, an immunotherapy drug developed by Merck Laboratories, which targets a molecular mechanism common to several cancers. Unlike previous treatments, Keytruda is effective against all tumors expressing the PD-1 protein, regardless of the tissues or organs affected.[20] The FDA's approval of such a targeted drug, allowing it to treat a subpopulation of patients defined by a molecular signature, has consecrated the advent of precision medicine as a therapeutic strategy of the future.

This concept of precision medicine is now extended by the pharmaceutical industry beyond oncology, for example, to neuropsychiatric, immune-inflammatory, respiratory, and metabolic diseases, which all have in common being very heterogeneous. It is also well suited to rare genetic diseases, of which only 5% currently have an effective treatment. To date, precision medicine represents only 5% of drug sales worldwide, but this figure could reach 20% in the years to come, particularly given the recent successes of gene therapy and the emergence of numerous molecular targeting modalities that we will discuss later.

Beyond that, a notable evolution is the increasingly frequent association of the drug with various "intelligent" medical devices that can assist in the prescription and dispensation of the drug. Medical devices are health products that are not sensu stricto drugs but include a variety of objects and applications that facilitate the use of drugs.[21] They include, for example, in vitro diagnostic tests as well as software and decision support algorithms for health professionals. These new tools allow biologists to interpret blood test results, doctors to refine their prescriptions, and pharmacists to check

[19] Trastuzumab® was marketed by the Roche laboratory as early as 1998, but its particularly remarkable effectiveness in patients with HER2+ breast cancer was demonstrated in 2005. Since 2012, Pfizer offers Xalkori® to treat 5% of patients with lung cancer, as long as they have a ROS1 gene mutation. The mutation of the KRAS oncogene allows to predict the effectiveness of Panitumumab, a drug based on anti-EGFR monoclonal antibody developed by the Amgen laboratory against metastatic colorectal cancer.

[20] This drug is prescribed to patients with melanoma, lung cancer, head and neck cancer, Hodgkin's disease, as long as the tumor cells express the PD-1 molecule.

[21] According to the definition of the Member States of the European Union, a medical device is defined as "*any instrument, device, equipment, material, product, excluding products of human origin, or other article used alone or in combination, including the accessories and software necessary for its proper functioning, intended by the manufacturer to be used in humans for medical purposes and whose main intended action is not achieved by pharmacological or immunological means or by metabolism, but whose function can be assisted by such means*".

drug compatibility before delivering treatments to patients. Some medical devices have a mechanical function and can be implanted in the human body, such as pacemakers, stents, prostheses, or even the first artificial organs. Many of these devices are qualified as "intelligent" as soon as they carry AI, allowing them to capture, transmit, and/or analyze data. These smart medical devices are considered complementary tools to drugs, to the point that they can even be physically associated with them. For example, a chip containing information about the identity and dose of the prescribed drug can be incorporated into the tablet at the same time as the active ingredient to confirm that the patient is taking their treatment correctly.[22]

In total, the new intelligence of a drug involves new approaches in its design, development, and use, made possible by AI. As we will see, AI will play a significant accelerator role in the evolution toward precision medicine, ensuring a perfect match between the understood characteristics of patients and the predicted properties of drugs. In synergy with advanced drug technologies, AI will be the engine of exponential drug innovation over the next few decades. And all the more so as the revolution now initiated by the intelligent drug is of great interest to a health industry capable of investing in research and development on a scale of billions of dollars…

Drug Innovation in a Knowledge Economy

As a driver of innovation, technologies play a central role in the global economy. In everyday language, the word technology refers to the application of advances in scientific knowledge to create new products, processes, or services that meet human needs. In a virtuous circle that feeds innovation, the sciences offer updated representations of the physical reality, also producing technological applications that allow us to act on the world as represented while accumulating new knowledge.[23]

[22] Medical devices are subject to a specific regulation, which tends to approach that of medicine. To be marketed in the European Union, a medical device must obtain a CE marking, attesting its compliance with safety and health standards defined by recent European directives. Medical devices are classified into 4 categories depending on their level of health risk, ranging from class 1 (low risk) to class 4 (highest risk). Each class is subject to specific evaluation and control rules. European regulations relating to medical devices were deeply revised in 2017 and came into force in 2021 for medical devices, and in 2022 for in vitro diagnostic medical devices. These new regulations aim to strengthen health safety and harmonize standards at the European level. Source: www.ansm.sante.fr. *ANSM: Nouveaux règlements européens relatifs aux dispositifs médicaux*, 2021. Specific regulations for medical devices using AI are currently being developed in Europe and the USA.

[23] See Rhodes and Wield [3] and Diamandis and Kotler [4]. According to Wikipedia, technology encompasses "*everything that can be said […] about the state of the art in terms of tools and know-how*". The word "technique" is commonly used to describe the way of doing something, that is, the processes used to produce and to achieve a specific result. In addition to health, new technologies open up enormous prospects in many fields, such as new materials, energy, transport, construction, communications, entertainment, electronics and of course computing. These technologies have considerable economic value on a societal scale and are often referred to as "defining" because they have the power to shape our relationship with the world. In the same vein, Francis Fukuyama highlighted in his essay on *The End of History and the Last Man* (Free Press, 2006), the political and structuring dimensions of technologies from a societal point of view.

The relationship between technology and the economy is not new. Economist Robin Hanson, a researcher at Oxford University, has highlighted the driving role in the global economy of technological disruptions observed throughout history, for example, during the agricultural revolution 5000 years ago or the industrial revolutions of the eighteenth and nineteenth centuries. The concept of a knowledge economy was attributed to Fritz Machlup, who described in those terms in 1962 an economy of knowledge and intangibles emerging at the time. In the 1990s, continuous technological advances led to the advent of "cognitive capitalism," marked notably by the emergence of digital giants in the United States, attracting huge investments and generating immense wealth. Alongside the digital, electronics, and automotive industries, health is one of the areas where private sector research and development (R&D) investments are most substantial.[24]

The health industry is therefore a central player in this knowledge economy, creating enormous societal wealth. The pursuit of profits in the health field is poorly perceived in some European countries, but it is much better accepted in the Anglo-Saxon world. We will see later that the costs associated with the development of a drug are typically on the order of several hundred million USD, or even more than USD 2.5 billion on average, to bring a new drug to market, if one takes into account the expenses associated with the many stopped projects. The need to make substantial profits is therefore essential for this industry, which continuously and at risk reinvests between 15% and 20% of its turnover in the development of new drugs.[25]

To explain such a substantial need for investment, it must also be remembered here that drug innovation has the particularities of an extremely long new product development cycle, characterized by great regulatory complexity and an extremely high failure rate. History confirms that, in the pharmaceutical field, more than 30 to 50 years, or even more, are frequently necessary to translate a new scientific concept into concrete applications, as summarized by Amara's law (see Box 2.1).

[24] According to the report Global Innovation 1000 by Price Waterhouse Cooper (B. Jaruzelski et al., *What the top innovators get right*) published in 2018, annual R&D investments in the private sector reached over $780 billion globally, across all sectors. Among the 20 companies investing more than $6 billion per year in R&D, we find digital and electronics players such as Amazon, Google's parent company Alphabet, Microsoft, Intel, Samsung, Apple, Facebook, Siemens, as well as health companies such as Roche, Johnson & Johnson, Merck, Novartis, Pfizer, Sanofi, and automotive industry players like Volkswagen, Toyota, Ford, General Motors, Daimler, Honda.

[25] According to IMS Health, the global pharmaceutical market has experienced significant growth in recent years, rising from $1010 billion in 2016 to $1161 billion in 2020, particularly thanks to drugs derived from biotechnologies. During this period, antiviral treatments accounted for about 15% of drug sales, followed by anticancer drugs (11%) and diabetes drugs (10%). Emerging countries accounted for about 75% of the growth in drug sales, compared to 17% for the United States and 6% for Europe. China is now the second largest pharmaceutical market with an estimated $180 billion in annual drug expenditures in 2020, behind the United States ($590 billion) and far ahead of France (sixth place with $38 billion). Source: Statista Research Department. *Pharmaceutical market: global turnover*. May 2022.

Box 2.1: Amara's Law: Praise of Perseverance

Major technological innovations generally follow three phases, as described in a "law" formulated by Roy Amara, founder of the Institute for the Future in Palo Alto, California. The first phase of innovation is marked by the enthusiasm that surrounds the emergence of a revolutionary idea resulting from recent scientific discoveries. The path from the concept to future applications initially seems clear, causing euphoria shared by researchers, investors, and future users. The second phase is that of pragmatism, when the difficulties encountered block or significantly slow down innovation, whose feasibility may even be doubted. The third phase is that of problem-solving, in which obstacles are gradually overcome and the achievements obtained sometimes exceed initial expectations! Roy Amara summarized these observations by reminding us how much we tend to overestimate the impact of a new technology in the short term and underestimate it in the long term![26]

Two examples among many others confirm that Amara's law applies to the discovery of new drugs, in which perseverance has proven indispensable to achieve success at the end of a long, winding road. Monoclonal antibodies (antibodies derived from a single cell clone produced in the laboratory, with a well-defined specificity), discovered by Georges Köhler and César Milstein in 1975, immediately raised hopes for future revolutionary drugs, given their ability to specifically recognize a precise target. After a period of euphoria, numerous difficulties were encountered, linked to undesirable immune responses and the complexity of their production. After more than 30 years of effort, monoclonal antibody-based drugs finally emerged, revolutionizing the treatment of many cancers and inflammatory diseases. These drugs now generate billions of dollars in annual sales worldwide, and their therapeutic applications continue to grow.

Similarly, gene therapy, which aims to replace or repair defective genes, was deemed revolutionary in the 1980s but seemed impossible 10 years later due to difficulties encountered during development. However, since the 2000s, young patients with rare genetic diseases have benefited from the first successes of gene therapy, radically transforming their prognosis. These drugs, now applied to an increasing number of diseases, have reached record prices, some exceeding several million dollars for a single injection!

[26] Amara's law finds echoes in the Gartner cycle (also called *hype cycle*), which reflects the different phases that accompany the maturation of technologies, before they produce first applications. The Gartner cycle distinguishes five phases in the life of a technology: the launch of innovation, followed by a peak of inflated expectations, then a trough of disillusionment, before reaching a phase of consolidation and a plateau of productivity.

Let us underline that Amara's law also applies to AI. The idea of designing machines that reproduce certain human cognitive abilities dates back to the middle of the twentieth century. After several "winters" linked to the limited computing power of computers at the time, but also to the lack of data and the absence of learning methods, AI has, in the last 10 years, reached the maturity necessary to transform all areas of human activity. AI has now entered the third phase of Amara's law, particularly with regard to applications in the field of health.

In the coming decades, three drivers of innovation will lead to an unprecedented acceleration in drug discovery. In addition to the virtuous cycle of investment in innovation/profit/reinvestment in new research, the needs of an aging human population for new drugs *(market pull)* will be combined with the technological opportunity linked to the meeting between AI and drug sciences *(technology push)*. It should be noted that investment in the discovery of intelligent drugs will certainly be acclaimed during the century by millennials and Generation Z, notoriously technophiles, as they will be confronted with age-related health problems. Collectively, these field forces invite us to anticipate unprecedented continuous and exponential innovation in the world of drugs, with the first signs of a dizzying revolution already perceptible, the multiple contours of which we shall now outline.

References

1. Dzau VJ, Fineberg HV, Shine KI, Thier SO, Morrissey S. A half century of progress in health. New Engl J Med. 2020;383:1293.
2. Strebhardt K, Ullrich A. Paul Ehrlich's magic bullet concept: 100 years of progress. Nat Rev Cancer. 2008;8:473.
3. Rhodes E, Wield D. Implementing new technologies. Milton Keynes: Open University Editions; 1994.
4. Diamandis P, Kotler S. Bold: how to go big, create wealth and impact the world. New York: Simon and Schuster; 2015.

3 Achievements and Promises of Biotechnologies

Genomics, Microbiota, and Drugs

Many innovative drug modalities stem from the continuous progress in genomics and molecular biology. An important turning point occurred at the dawn of the new millennium with the sequencing of the human genome. By the end of the twentieth century, decisive improvements in DNA sequencing technologies had made it possible to analyze the genomes of many species, whether bacteria, plants, or higher animals. In 2003, the publication of the first complete sequence of the human genome, assembled from multiple donors, paved the way for a better understanding of our genetic heritage. This sequencing carried out by the *Human Genome Project* consortium required 15 years of effort and cost USD 2.7 billion, as it was based on the non-automated Sanger method. With the advent of next-generation DNA and RNA sequencing technologies, the sequencing of a human genome can now be performed robotically in a few hours for a cost of about USD 1000, or even USD 600 if focused on the exome, that is, the part of the DNA that codes for proteins.[1]

During this decryption of the human genome, the excitement was at its peak, as humanity was going to be able to contemplate its genetic heritage "as in an open book" (see Box 3.1).

[1] In 1996, the laboratories of the Genopole in Évry, France, carried out the first mapping of the organization of the human genome, locating many genes on the 23 pairs of chromosomes that make up our genome. The first complete sequencing of the human genome was carried out by the international scientific collaboration *Human Genome Project*, in competition with the biotechnology company Celera Genomics, founded by American researcher Craig Venter. The first complete genome from a single individual was sequenced in 2007.

P. Moingeon, *Intelligent Drugs: How AI is Transforming Healthcare*,
https://doi.org/10.1007/978-3-031-91668-7_3

Box 3.1:What Have We Learned from Sequencing the Human Genome?
Sequencing a genome involves determining the order of the molecular bricks called nucleotides, which make up our DNA. This macromolecule is presented in the form of two strands wound into a double helix that contains our genes, inherited from each parent, located inside our chromosomes. The human genome includes about 23,000 genes coding for 30,000 proteins.

The analysis of the human genome has deepened our understanding of the molecular processes characterizing the human being. While highlighting a common heritage to humanity, the sequencing of multiple genomes has demonstrated the extraordinary variability of our species at the biological level and, beyond that, the uniqueness of each individual.[2] It also allowed a better understanding of diseases, thus giving a new impetus to biotechnologies and their applications in the manipulation of the living, with many drugs targeting biological processes now better understood. Genomic sequencing, which is becoming more common, has allowed the identification of genetic susceptibility loci to hundreds of diseases, thus opening the door to predictive molecular diagnosis and to gene therapy, which aims to replace a defective gene.

In the years that followed, research has highlighted the complex workings of information transmission in the living world, far from being reduced to a simple correspondence between a gene and a protein. It has been established that this transmission involves gene expression regulation mechanisms operating at the levels of DNA (epigenetic modifications), RNA (*editing*), and protein (post-translational modifications[3]).

Beyond the sequencing of the human genome, two other major discoveries have illuminated the complex interaction between genes and the environment over the past 15 years. The first discovery concerns epigenetics, a research field that has recently revealed that the DNA that makes up the genes in our cells can undergo chemical modifications induced by our relationship to the environment and our lifestyle (diet, stress, smoking, and other addictions). These epigenetic modifications,

[2] It is indeed forbidden to patent genes or DNA sequences that are part of this heritage unique to our species, patent protection being only possible for applications designed from this knowledge.

[3] The transmission of information within the cell is based on the transcription of DNA (deoxyribonucleic acid) into RNA (ribonucleic acid), followed by the translation of RNA into proteins. Chemical modifications of DNA, called epigenetic modifications, influence gene expression. These modifications, for example in the form of DNA methylation or acetylation of proteins called histones that structure DNA, are induced reversibly or persistently by our relationship with the environment. In addition, messenger RNAs can be modified and regulated by other RNAs such as microRNAs. Proteins, after their translation into amino acids, can undergo chemical modifications (glycosylation, phosphorylation, sialylation…) that affect their half-life and their biological function. All these regulatory mechanisms introduce a relative plasticity in the DNA, RNA and proteins relationship during the transmission of intra-cellular information.

which can be passed on to the offspring, do not alter the nucleotide sequence of the genes but can impact their expression. They explain why monozygotic twins, who have a rigorously identical genetic heritage, can present differences in their observable characteristics.

Meanwhile, another discovery revealed that humans have a "second genome"! This genome comes from our microbiota, that is to say, all the microorganisms, mainly bacteria, that colonize our digestive tract and our respiratory or genital mucosae. The terms "microbiota" and "microbiome" are used to describe, respectively, the microorganisms themselves or their genomes.[4] With more than 10^{13} bacteria colonizing each human being, it is estimated that the number of genes expressed by the microbiota is nearly a hundred times greater than that of all the cells in our body combined![5] Like epigenetic modifications, the composition of this microbiota is also influenced by our lifestyle habits and our diet, as well as our age and the medications we take. All this knowledge about our genetic heritage and the interaction between our genes and the environment has proven very useful for the design of new drugs. The deciphering of the human genome has indeed made it possible to better understand the influence of certain genes on the response to drugs, leading to the birth of a new discipline, pharmacogenomics. This has highlighted the many genes involved in the absorption, metabolism (mainly at the liver level), and excretion of drugs, as well as their significant variability within the human population. In addition, the crucial role in health played by the mechanisms of epigenetics was quickly confirmed, as some of the chemical modifications of DNA related to an individual's experience can confer on their offspring a risk of cardiovascular diseases, obesity, or cancers. We have also discovered the very important role of the microbiota in the metabolism of our food, but also that of drugs, contributing to the proper functioning of our immune system. Recent research suggests that a low diversity of the microbiota at the mucosal level can promote the onset of many diseases, a discovery opening the field to new preventive or therapeutic approaches.

All these scientific advances have proven crucial for better understanding individual variations in terms of predisposition to diseases and response to drugs. This knowledge has made it possible to treat certain diseases caused by genetic mutations using gene therapy, which we will discuss below. Other drugs, now in clinical evaluation, target the epigenetic modifications of certain genes responsible for

[4] Our first genome is composed of DNA containing genes located in the chromosomes of our cells. Most of the bacteria in our microbiota, known as commensals, are harmless, they limit the proliferation of pathogenic bacteria. The term "microbiota" refers to all microorganisms present in a specific environment and includes bacteria, viruses, and fungi.

[5] According to estimates, our body would carry 1 to 10 times more bacteria than human cells. These figures do not, however, take into account the many viruses, phages, and fungi that we host. Considering that a human carries about 1000 bacterial species in his gut, each possessing an average of 2000 genes, the intestinal bacterial microbiota enriches us with two million genes (or 90 times more than those that make up the human genome), endowed with their own functions many of which are useful to our species!

cancers. At the same time, new therapeutic approaches are exploring the manipulation of patients' microbiota, as well as the development of drugs from the molecules secreted by the bacteria that make up our second genome. The first microbiota-based drug, Robyota®, was thus approved in 2022 by the FDA to prevent the recurrence of severe infectious diarrhea.[6]

In summary, these new scientific insights at the dawn of the third millennium have allowed us to understand that there are considerable variations in the human population in terms of genetic heritage, as well as gene-environment interactions, resulting in significant differences, depending on the individual, in responses to drugs. These insights have proven fundamental in encouraging the design of precision medicine based on more personalized treatments. With to further progress to this aim, unprecedented possibilities for a detailed characterization of the human at the molecular level.

Molecular Profiling of Humans

Interest in the human genome has promoted the large-scale use of high-throughput DNA and RNA sequencing technologies, particularly to understand interindividual variations in genomic sequences and their possible link with different diseases. These variations often take the form of simple point modifications at the DNA level (called SNPs, pronounced [snips] for *single-nucleotide polymorphisms*). These have been the subject of extensive research, listing more than 70,000 associations between SNPs and human phenotypic characteristics to date.[7] Some companies, like the California-based 23andMe, already market tests for genetic susceptibility to certain diseases based on the detection of mutations or polymorphisms in DNA sequences. These tests are performed on saliva samples to predict the risk of developing diseases such as diabetes, breast cancer, Alzheimer's disease, or various cardiovascular diseases.[8] In practice, however, their interpretation remains delicate, as

[6] Therapeutic manipulations of microbiota are the subject of numerous clinical studies in various diseases. Some approaches involve administering extracts of fecal matter from healthy subjects to people suffering from recurrent infections to *Clostridium difficile* (a bacterium causing severe diarrhea), thus restoring a normal intestinal flora. Other fecal transplantation approaches of microbiota from melanoma patients who respond favorably to immunotherapy are currently being studied to treat non-responding patients. In the future, bacterial transplants will be replaced by the administration of bacteria grown in the laboratory, thus offering treatments of controlled pharmaceutical quality. Robyota® is the first drug of this new therapeutic class, composed of several bacterial strains isolated from the fecal flora of healthy subjects. Eventually, drugs could be developed from the molecules secreted by these bacteria that have an interesting therapeutic activity, for example in the regulation of the immune system, to avoid inflammatory reactions.

[7] https://www.ebi.ac.uk/gwas/

[8] These genetic tests, which cost a few hundred dollars, are performed from oral epithelial cells collected by simple scraping of the inside of the cheek with a cotton swab.

often hundreds of genetic variants contribute to determining susceptibility to a disease. Moreover, many patients do not wish to be informed of genetic predispositions to diseases for which there is no effective treatment, such as Alzheimer's or Huntington's. Faced with a test revealing a statistical risk—and not an absolute certainty—of developing cancer or another disease in the future, the behavior to adopt, beyond increased surveillance, remains a complex question.[9]

Beyond these genetic tests, remarkable progress in the biomedical diagnosis targeting proteins has been made over the past 20 years, for example, with the development of self-tests performed by the patient or rapid diagnostic orientation tests implemented by a health professional. These tests make it easy to detect pregnancy, diabetes, or certain viral or bacterial infections. Automation and robotization have also improved the reliability, speed, and productivity of biological tests performed routinely in centralized laboratories.[10] At the same time, advances have allowed the development of miniaturized and sensitive tests, opening the way for multiplex analysis, that is, the simultaneous measurement of several biological parameters from a single blood sample. In a scandal that recently made headlines, the Californian biotech company Theranos aimed to develop a diagnostic test combining the measurement of 10,000 biological parameters from a simple drop of blood taken from the fingertip, all for a cost of less than USD 3![11] While Theranos proved unable to keep its promises, miniaturized multiparametric protein tests retain all their interest, with the goal of extending the scope of current routine biological assessments while controlling their costs. Indeed, the possibility of performing a comprehensive molecular diagnosis from a drop of blood appears realistic today thanks to the rapid evolution of molecular typing technologies. The use of antibodies coupled with "tags" of DNA, combined with high-throughput DNA sequencing to read these tags, now allows us to envisage the parallel quantification of 3000 proteins from a single microliter of blood![12]

---

[9] For these reasons, these genetic tests are not authorized in France. cf. the report of the French National Ethics Advisory Committee (CCNE) published in 2016: "*Réflexion éthique sur l'évolution des tests génétiques liée au séquençage de l'ADN humain à très haut débit*". The French Senate, however, adopted in 2018 a bill authorizing their use for deceased persons, justifying this decision by the potential interest for the close family, in terms of medical follow-up.

[10] These routine biological analyses commonly include a blood ionogram and a blood cell count, supplemented as needed by more specific dosages to assess the metabolism of glucose or lipids, or by dosages of hormones or biomarkers associated with a particular biological function.

[11] Theranos was a biotechnology company founded in 2003, which generated considerable interest, reaching a valuation of $9 billion US on the stock market. Its leader Elisabeth Holmes had managed to convince several Silicon Valley personalities to invest in her project rightly considered revolutionary. However, Theranos only managed to develop a very limited number of dosages with uncertain results, and it subcontracted most of its analyses to external companies performing the dosages with traditional methods! This scandal was revealed by John Carreyrou in his book *Bad blood: Theranos scandal, secrets and lies at the heart of Silicon Valley*. Vintage Edition, 2018. The company was dissolved at the end of 2018 and Elisabeth Holmes was convicted of fraud in 2022.

[12] This approach is currently being studied on 50,000 individuals as part of the *Pharma Proteomics project*. UK Biobank. Pharma Proteomics Project. https://www.ukbiobank.ac.uk/

In addition to routine diagnostic methods, there are other molecular profiling technologies called "multi-omics," which are used for research purposes to establish the detailed characteristics of an individual, healthy or sick, from a blood or tissue sample. These approaches include—in addition to genome sequencing—transcriptomics, metabolomics, and proteomics, which, respectively, allow us to quantify the gene expression, analyze metabolism-related molecules, and characterize the majority of proteins. Transcriptomic and proteomic analyses can even now be conducted in parallel on individual cells![13]

Today, these in-depth multi-omics analyses are commonly performed on biological samples from a few dozen or a hundred patients participating in clinical studies to evaluate new drugs. They are not yet routinely offered for diagnostic purposes due to the high costs and complexity associated with analyzing the enormous amounts of data generated. However, it is not excluded that these technologies could, within a decade, gradually supplement or even replace current blood tests to qualitatively and quantitatively characterize the biological specificities of each individual, from simple blood samples or small tissue or tumor biopsies.[14]

We will further explore the remarkable complementarity of these molecular profiling technologies, which provide large amounts of biological data, and AI, which allows the interpretation of these massive and varied data. We will see that high-resolution medical imaging technologies also provide a considerable amount of data on the patient's health status, which is efficiently exploitable thanks to AI. The availability of detailed data on the characteristics of each patient, as well as healthy individuals, combined with their analysis by AI, will be a significant driver of the intelligent drug revolution.

---

[13] Specifically, coupled with genome sequencing and epigenetic analyses, transcriptomics allows, thanks to high-throughput sequencing of messenger RNAs, to quantify the expression of 23,000 genes; metabolomics analyzes several hundred molecules reflecting major metabolisms, whereas proteomics documents the expression of thousands of proteins. Proteomics and metabolomics use mass spectrometry, a method allowing to identify molecules by very precisely determining their mass. By combining these approaches with histological examinations consisting of the microscopic analysis of biopsies or surgical samples, researchers are now trying to reconstruct in 3D, at the molecular and cellular level, the biological processes related to a disease in a tissue or an organ. This technology of "spatial" molecular profiling was elected technology of the year in 2020 by the journal *Nature*.

[14] In parallel, a recent development in oncology involves diagnosing certain solid tumors from blood samples assimilated to liquid biopsies, less invasive than tissue biopsies, by detecting the fragments of DNA released by tumor cells into the blood. A comparable approach is used to screen for chromosomal abnormalities of the fetus during pregnancy, notably trisomy 21, by analyzing the DNA of rare fetal cells circulating in the maternal blood, thus avoiding an invasive procedure such as amniocentesis.

A Booming Gene Therapy

Gene therapy is one of the great successes of post-genomic medicine. It addresses diseases caused by the inactivation or dysfunction of a gene, for example, following a mutation. Several forms of gene therapy are available or in development, but the most classic approach is to reintroduce a functional copy of the altered gene into the patient using a vector, usually a non-pathogenic virus for humans. This recombinant viral vector carries the normal human gene like a Trojan horse into the patient's cells, allowing the production of the missing protein and thus restoring the altered biological function.[15]

Currently, gene therapy is limited to so-called monogenic diseases, which involve a single gene, such as certain immune deficiencies, rare metabolic diseases, or blood diseases. Genetic diseases in which several genes are involved are not yet accessible to this therapy. Another challenge is the immune response that the viral vector elicits in the patient, which can limit the treatment to a single administration by reducing its long-term effectiveness.

Despite the obstacles encountered over the decades, the expected benefits of gene therapy have finally been confirmed, notably by revolutionizing the treatment of certain rare diseases with a new class of drugs (see Box 3.2).

Box 3.2: The First Successes of Gene Therapy

Since the 1980s, gene therapy has attracted the interest of researchers in light of advances in molecular biology, allowing the envisioning of gene transfer methods. However, the death of a patient during a clinical study in 1999 in the United States almost compromised its future. A major turning point in the early 2000s was the success of gene therapy in treating severe immune deficiencies in "bubble babies," achieved by Professor Alain Fischer's team at the Necker Hospital in Paris.[16]

Since then, impressive clinical results have been obtained in other genetic diseases, saving the lives of patients with rare diseases previously incurable (adenosine deficiency, X-linked adrenoleukodystrophy, or Wiskott-Aldrich syndrome). The American and European health agencies have recognized the innovative nature of these approaches, authorizing the use of these drugs to

(continued)

[15] The viruses used are lentiviruses, adenoviruses, or adeno-associated viruses which are not dangerous to humans, but which effectively infect human cells. We speak of recombinant virus to designate these genetically modified viruses to insert into their nucleotide sequence the gene to be restored.

[16] The patients are very young boys affected by a severe combined immune deficiency linked to the X chromosome. These children whose immune defenses are greatly weakened are nicknamed "bubble babies", as they must be confined in a controlled environment to be protected from infections.

Box 3.2 (continued)

treat an increasing number of severe pathologies without a therapeutic alternative. Gene therapy has thus been established as a therapeutic modality for rare diseases, sometimes even adapted to individual cases, as we will illustrate later.

A hurdle to gene therapy remains to this day the large-scale production of recombinant viruses carrying the gene to be repaired while respecting the pharmaceutical quality required for any drug. This bottleneck has been partially lifted by the emergence of several specialized biotechnology companies in the USA, such as Spark Therapeutics, BioMarin, and Bluebird Bio, but also in Europe with UniQure, Yposkesi, and Cellectis. Due to the significant investments required for the industrial production of complex gene therapy treatments, the cost of these new drugs is high, averaging one million euros per treated patient.

The long-awaited success of gene therapy was celebrated as a revolution in the health industry forum organized by JP Morgan in San Francisco in January 2019, arousing great interest among pharmaceutical giants with considerable investment capacities.

The first successes of gene therapy in extremely rare diseases have been confirmed by several developments in new indications. In 2015, a study showed that the introduction of the RPE65 gene restored the sight of patients suffering from retinitis pigmentosa, a genetic disease causing progressive blindness.[17]

More recently, a gene therapy product, Zolgensma®, has shown its effectiveness in spinal muscular atrophy, a rare, progressive, and hitherto fatal disease. This treatment is now among the most expensive in the world because, even though it only requires a single injection, its cost is 1.9 million €! Moreover, gene therapy has recently also proven to be effective in the treatment of more common blood diseases, such as hemophilia A and B, sickle cell disease, and beta-thalassemia, significantly improving the condition of patients after a single administration of the vectorized healthy gene. In particular, the FDA authorized the marketing in 2022 of Zynteglo®, a gene therapy drug based on a lentivirus carrying the normal beta-globin gene to treat patients suffering from major beta-thalassemia, a disease that required regular red blood cell transfusions until now. In the same year, the American agency also approved Hemgenix®, an adeno-associated virus restoring the expression of the normal gene coding for clotting factor IX in patients suffering from

[17] An obstacle to widespread use in this disease, which illustrates a limit to which gene therapy remains faced, is that several hundred genes are involved in retinitis pigmentosa. Mutations in the RPE65 gene only concern 2% of patients with this disease.

hemophilia B.[18] In the spring of 2024, Lenmeldy®, a gene therapy drug developed by Orchard Therapeutics, was registered in the United States to treat patients suffering from metachromatic leukodystrophy. At 4.25 million US dollars per injection, it is currently the most expensive drug in the world!

Alongside the use of recombinant viruses, a new form of gene therapy is generating great interest for the treatment of certain cancers. This approach involves administering the patient's own immune cells after their modification in the laboratory. T lymphocytes are first isolated from the patient's blood and then infected with a virus that transfers a receptor (called CAR) to them, allowing them to effectively recognize and kill tumor cells. These modified immune cells, known as *CAR T cells*, are then reinjected into the patient. Kymriah® was the first gene therapy based on *CAR T cells* to be authorized in the United States in 2017.[19] Today, genetically modified T lymphocytes are used to treat certain leukemias or lymphomas, with spectacular results, leading to regressions and complete remissions in more than half of the patients. For some patients, this therapy has eradicated tumor cells in the blood for over 10 years, suggesting a real cure. This is a particularly remarkable result, as many of these blood cancers were previously resistant to all existing treatments! To broaden the scope of this type of drug, the use of *CAR T cells* is currently being explored in patients with solid tumors. However, this approach remains complex, as it requires laboratory manipulation of each treated patient's immune cells.[20]

It took 40 years for gene therapy to produce a new class of drugs that have radically transformed the prognosis of many diseases. The production and high cost of these complex drugs are now a significant limit to their large-scale use. Despite this, tens of new gene therapy drugs are expected by 2030, posing a challenge to health systems in managing the cost of these treatments intended for a limited number of patients. Strengthened by its initial successes, gene therapy now benefits from the emergence of specialized biotech companies, recognition by regulatory authorities, and the growing interest of large pharmaceutical companies in these drugs applicable to an increasing range of genetic diseases. Moreover, gene therapy is experiencing an additional boost with new technologies, in the form of molecular scissors, allowing the design of unprecedented targeted drugs.

---

[18] Hemgenix® is administered by a single intravenous infusion. In the case of Zynteglo®, patients are treated with their own hematopoietic stem cells (capable of producing blood cells), previously infected in the laboratory by the lentiviral vector carrying the healthy beta-globin gene. These treated patients are then able to produce normal hemoglobin over time, necessary for the production of red blood cells. Magrin et al. [1].

[19] T lymphocytes are central cells in the functioning of the immune system. In particular, one of their functions is to recognize and destroy tumor cells or cells infected by viruses. CAR is the abbreviation for *chimeric antigen receptor*, to designate the chimeric receptor capable of recognizing a target protein expressed by tumor cells. The *CAR T cells* of the Kymriah® type produced by the Novartis laboratory have also been used in Europe since 2019.

[20] An alternative approach studied in humans consists in treating patients with the same line of *CAR T cells*, called allogeneic, easier to produce on an industrial scale.

Molecular Targeting of All Kinds

As we have seen, an interesting property of intelligent drugs is that they are specifically directed against a therapeutic target selected on the basis of a solid scientific rationale. Thanks to the emerging new therapeutic modalities, we can now target the active principle of drugs at different molecular levels of DNA, RNA, or protein.

In addition to the gene therapy approaches previously mentioned, methods of modifying DNA allow the insertion or deletion of entire genes or specific fragments at precise locations in nucleotide sequences. These so-called *gene editing* tools are designed based on enzymes (such as CRISPR-Cas9, the *zinc finger nucleases* or ZFNs, and the *transcription activator-like effector nucleases* or TALENs) to make targeted cuts in DNA. The cellular machinery then naturally repairs these cuts, with frequent insertions or deletions of nucleotides that inactivate the targeted gene. Conversely, it is also possible to restore the function of the gene by inserting an intact copy at the site of the cut. Among these methods, the molecular scissors designed in 2016 from the bacterial enzyme CRISPR-Cas9 generated particular interest, as it allows easy editing of any nucleotide base in the genome.[21] This technology earned the 2020 Nobel Prize in Chemistry for American Jennifer Doudna and Frenchwoman Emmanuelle Charpentier. Today, it is commonly used in research laboratories to "cut and paste" pieces of DNA as well as to inactivate or modify a specific gene.

Clinical studies have quickly evaluated treatments using these targeted genome modification technologies to correct mutations causing various genetic diseases. It is estimated today that over a hundred clinical studies have been conducted or are in progress that use the CRISPR-Cas9 technology to treat different types of cancers as well as blood diseases [2, 3]. Several research teams are thus modifying the genome of T lymphocytes from patients with melanoma, sarcoma (soft tissue cancer), multiple myeloma (bone marrow cancer), and lung cancer in order to restore their immunity against tumor cells. The modification made here consists of deleting the PD-1 gene in the immune cells so that the tumor cells can no longer inhibit them. In parallel, other research focuses on the manipulation using CRISPR-Cas9 of hematopoietic stem cells from patients with sickle cell disease or beta-thalassemia so that they can produce normal hemoglobin. By the end of 2023, Casgevy® became the first CRISPR-Cas9-based drug authorized by the regulatory agencies of Great Britain and the United States to treat patients with sickle cell disease, with the prospect of a real cure. These genetic manipulations in adults suffering from serious diseases do not affect reproductive cells, thus avoiding any ethical problem. However, the recent use of CRISPR-Cas9 by a Chinese researcher to alter the genome of human embryos has sparked strong reactions in the scientific community

[21] CRISPR is an acronym for frequently repeated nucleotide sequences in DNA. CRISPR-Cas9 is a natural enzymatic system used by bacteria to destroy the genetic material of viruses and phages that infect them.

due to the transmissible nature of these modifications to the future offspring of these embryos.

Other drugs target RNAs using oligonucleotides, that is, small molecules composed of about 20 chemically synthesized nucleotides. These oligonucleotides bind specifically to target RNAs, allowing for the increase or inhibition of the expression of the genes of interest. When the oligonucleotide inhibits a defective gene coding for an abnormal protein, we speak of *gene silencing*. Two antisense oligonucleotide-based drugs, Spinraza® and Tofersen®, have recently been registered to treat patients with neurological diseases affecting the neurons controlling the muscles, especially respiratory ones. This approach seems promising for treating other neurological diseases, such as Parkinson's or Huntington's disease, as well as forms of currently incurable muscle degeneration, such as Duchenne muscular dystrophy, or even certain cancers. Notably, these methods of targeting DNAs by editing approaches or RNAs by synthetic oligonucleotides are considered forms of gene therapy.[22]

Finally, numerous drug approaches specifically targeting proteins are currently being explored. We have already mentioned monoclonal antibodies, acting as *magic bullets*, which today constitute the active ingredients of more than 70 drugs, collectively generating over USD 125 billion in annual sales worldwide. Other promising developments are underway, such as bispecific antibodies capable of recognizing two proteins simultaneously, as well as antibodies conjugated to drug molecules—for example, chemotherapies—to specifically target certain tissues or cells. A dozen bispecific antibodies have been marketed to date to treat different cancers, and about 50 are currently under clinical evaluation in humans. A total of 13 drugs combining an antibody with chemotherapy are already authorized to treat different blood cancers or solid tumors.[23]

In addition to monoclonal antibodies, new therapeutic approaches aim to specifically degrade abnormal proteins, either due to mutations, overproduction, or modifications in their three-dimensional structure. Several drug candidates are under study, consisting of a specific recognition module of the protein to be degraded, combined with another module allowing the addition of a degradation signal to the targeted protein.[24] This targeted approach to the degradation of abnormal proteins is particularly interesting in age-related neurodegenerative diseases, in which

[22] High and Roncarolo [4]. Nusinersen (Spinraza®) used in the treatment of spinal muscular atrophy is designed to activate the SMN2 gene and produce the corresponding protein, essential for the survival of motor neurons. Tofersen® inhibits the RNA coding for the SOD1 protein mutated in some patients with amyotrophic lateral sclerosis, causing the death of motor neurons. Administration to patients at an early stage of Huntington's disease of an oligonucleotide inhibiting the messenger RNA coding for a toxic protein, huntingtin, has reduced the expression of this protein responsible for the disease.

[23] Ecker et al. [5]. Bispecific antibodies have two arms that recognize two distinct antigens, for example carried respectively by tumor cells and by immune cells, in order to activate the latter.

[24] This second module recruits an enzyme that adds a ubiquitin molecule to the targeted protein. This acts as a powerful signal for destruction by the cellular machinery.

aggregates of abnormal proteins induce neuronal death. It is also being studied to destroy abnormal proteins in patients with cancer or to target proteins involved in cellular aging, thus paving the way for the first anti-aging drugs, as we will see.

Drugs Produced by Plants and Animals

Biotechnologies allow the modification of living organisms by gene transfer in order to confer new properties on them. We will focus here on the transformation of plants and animals to make them produce drug molecules. Since antiquity, humans have practiced the selection and crossbreeding of species through agriculture and livestock breeding, mainly for food reasons. These traditional methods of genetic mixing are, however, slow and limited compared to current technologies, which allow DNA to be modified in a few days, or even a few hours, in the form of mutations, deletions, and gene insertions.

Today, the genetic modification of plants is commonly used to increase their resistance to pests or pesticides, stimulate their growth, and improve their nutritional value, thus contributing to increasing crop productivity. Genetically modified organisms (GMOs) are considered by many experts as essential to address world hunger, which still affects nearly one billion people.[25] About 10% of cultivated land worldwide, or more than 180 million hectares, is currently used to produce genetically modified plants, such as soybeans and corn (representing together 80% of GMO crops), but also cotton and rapeseed.

The genetic modification of plants that interests us here is the one that is called *molecular farming* (or *pharming*). It consists of inserting human genes into plants to produce large quantities of therapeutic proteins with a natural three-dimensional structure and is intended, as such, to serve as the basis for drugs. It has the advantage of avoiding any risk of transmission of infectious agents to patients, unlike the direct use of materials of human or animal origin. Human growth hormone was the first drug protein produced in a transgenic plant in 1986. Other proteins of medical interest obtained from plant transgenesis include erythropoietin, albumin, interferon α, certain toxins, various allergens, vaccine antigens, and monoclonal antibodies. The plant species commonly used to produce these drugs are tobacco, tomatoes, corn, potatoes, and rice. All these plants have in common the ability to allow large-scale cultivation and easy purification of the therapeutic protein from plant tissues. Even for a medical application, the creation of such GMOs is not always well accepted by the population. As an example, in 2005, transgenic corn crops carried

[25] In developed countries, the prospect of intensive agriculture and the use of GMOs to increase agricultural production are unpopular. However, as Thomas Robert Malthus pointed out as early as 1798 in his essay on *The Principle of Population*, improving agricultural productivity is critical in the fight against global hunger. Selective crops, the use of fertilizers, phytosanitary products and more recently GMOs aim to increase agricultural production to feed a global population of 8 billion individuals.

out in France by the company Meristem to produce a gastric lipase were thus destroyed by anti-GMO activists.[26]

Genetically modified animals are also used to meet food or medical needs. Genetic selection of livestock has also been practiced for a long time by humanity, with animal breeding now guided by very advanced scientific knowledge. Gene *editing* technologies, such as CRISPR-Cas-9 or TALEN, are commonly used to directly modify the genome of animals. While many of these applications aim to improve the quality of meat from livestock, an American biotechnology company plans to create hypoallergenic cats by inactivating the gene coding for the main feline allergen, called Fel d 1. These GMO animals will eventually be destined for cat lovers who are predisposed to severe allergic reactions in their presence! Moreover, the use of genetically modified animals is particularly useful for biomedical research in order to evaluate new drugs in the laboratory. For about 30 years, it has been possible to create in the laboratory transgenic animals, mutants, *knock-outs,* or *knock-ins* for specific genes—typically mice or rats—thus offering numerous disease models aiming to replicate those of humans. As we will see later, these models are commonly used to study the effectiveness and toxicity of drug candidates in the laboratory before evaluating them in humans.[27]

The genetic modification of animals to produce drugs, called *farmaceuticals*, is a practice similar to that used for plants. For example, human genes are added to animals such as goats or rabbits to make them produce therapeutic proteins in their milk. The first drug obtained in this way was Atryn®, an anticoagulant produced in the milk of genetically modified goats, which was approved for use in humans in the United States in 2009. Another drug, Ruconest®, marketed since 2014 to treat hereditary angioedema (a form of hives that affects deep tissues), is produced from the milk of transgenic rabbits. In 2015, the FDA also authorized the marketing of Kanuma®, a drug to treat a rare metabolic disease whose active principle is a human enzyme produced in the eggs of genetically modified chickens.[28]

Other research involves the genetic modification of animals to provide transplantable organs for humans. Xenotransplantation, that is, the grafting of animal organs to humans, was explored in the 1990s, mainly using pigs and sows, because

[26] Gastric lipase was considered as the active ingredient of a drug to treat patients with cystic fibrosis. An alternative to GMOs is to produce therapeutic proteins from laboratory cultures of plant cells transfected with the gene of interest. This approach allows for more controlled confinement than the cultivation of GMO plants in the field, but production yields are more limited.

[27] The laboratory animals used are mice or rats in which a gene has been specifically introduced (transgenic animal) or on the contrary deleted (knock-out animal), or replaced by another gene (knock-in animal), the rest of the animal's genetic heritage remaining unchanged.

[28] Atryn® is a recombinant human antithrombin. After giving a favorable opinion on its use in humans in 2006, the European agency EMA subsequently requested the addition of a filtration step during production, in view of the strict safety measures imposed on products of animal origin since the mad cow disease crisis. Ruconest®, authorized in the USA and Europe, is a C1-esterase inhibitor. Kanuda® is used to treat patients suffering from a deficiency in lysosomal acid lipase, a disease that causes an accumulation of fats in the liver, spleen and cardiovascular system.

the size of their organs (especially the heart and kidney) is close to that of humans. These approaches were, however, abandoned due to the problems of rejection of an organ of animal origin and also the risk of transmission of pig viruses to humans. Today, there is a renewed interest in xenotransplantation, combined with genetic modifications of animals to inactivate viruses naturally infecting pigs but also minimize the risk of rejection of the animal graft.[29]

Finally, in a completely different application, the American companies Oxitec and Mosquito Mate are working on the genetic modification of Asian tiger mosquitoes of the species *Aedes (A. albopictus and A. aegypti)*, known to transmit dangerous viral infections to humans. These genetically modified mosquitoes are designed as a "treatment" to combat the hemorrhagic fevers spread by these insects. By rendering them sterile, they indeed prevent wild mosquitoes from reproducing in nature. In the southern United States and Brazil, these sterile Aedes mosquitoes have been experimentally released to limit the spread of dengue and Zika viruses by wild insects. If this strategy proves effective, it could also reduce the transmission of chikungunya and yellow fever viruses. This approach could also be extended to the genetic modification of the mosquito *Anopheles gambiae* by making it resistant to the parasite responsible for malaria, which causes 230 million infections each year and results in more than 400,000 deaths worldwide.[30]

[29]The team of Georges Church, Professor at the Harvard Medical School, in collaboration with the company eGenesis, are pioneering second-generation xenotransplantation. They recently implanted human stem cells into pig embryos to obtain chimeric animals with "humanized" organs, which could be better tolerated by patients awaiting transplantation.

[30]The impact of the large-scale release of genetically modified insects on ecosystems is currently being studied, it should be limited because these insects released into the wild are unable to reproduce.

References

1. Magrin E, et al. Long-term outcomes of lentiviral gene therapy for the b-hemoglobinopathies: the hgb-205 trial. Nature Med. 2022;28:81.
2. Zhang S, et al. Current trends in clinical trials involving CRISPR/Cas systems. Front Med. 2023;10:1292452.
3. Sheridan C. The world's first CRISPR therapy is approved: who will receive it? Nature Biotechnol. 2024;42:3.
4. High KA, Roncarolo MC. Gene therapy. New Engl J Med. 2019;381:455.
5. Ecker D, et al. The therapeutic monoclonal antibody market. mAbs. 2015;7:9.

4 Breakthrough Therapeutic Modalities

Stem Cells and Regenerative Medicine

At the embryonic stage, the human body is rich in pluripotent stem cells, which are capable of transforming into the different types of cells that make up the body. The concept of regenerative medicine is based on the use of these cells to repair failing or aging organs. For a long time, the only source of such cells was the embryo, which obviously raised important ethical questions. In 2012, Japanese researcher Shinya Yamanaka overcame this ethical barrier by obtaining pluripotent stem cells from simple adult subject cells. By introducing certain genes into adult mouse skin cells, he managed to transform them into induced pluripotent stem cells (iPSCs). This breakthrough has opened up real prospects in regenerative medicine, as iPSCs can be obtained from the patient's own cells, thus avoiding not only the use of embryos but also problems of immunogenicity and rejection. Specialized companies have been able to offer wealthy individuals the production of such stem cells in the laboratory by reprogramming their skin cells. The stem cells thus obtained can then be stored for use in the treatment of future diseases.

However, 13 years after Professor Yamanaka's Nobel Prize-winning discovery, the therapeutic applications of stem cells are still awaited. Although scientific knowledge in this field has advanced considerably, the use of pluripotent progenitor cells remains complex. The very first trials of administration in humans of muscle or cardiac cells derived from stem cells were stopped, as they required at the time the use of cells from human embryos. The first clinical trial with iPSCs was conducted in 2015 at the Riken Institute for Developmental Biology in Japan. These researchers used induced pluripotent stem cells derived from the skin of a patient suffering from blindness due to age-related macular degeneration. They thus obtained in the laboratory pigmented cells from the retinal epithelium, which they reinjected into the patient. Although retinal degeneration was halted, the treatment had to be stopped due to genetic mutations detected in the administered cells.

P. Moingeon, *Intelligent Drugs: How AI is Transforming Healthcare*,
https://doi.org/10.1007/978-3-031-91668-7_4

Despite these difficulties, research in regenerative medicine continues actively. Researchers have learned to modify these stem cells by adding or removing certain genes using the *gene-editing* techniques mentioned earlier. Hundreds of clinical trials with iPSC cells have been conducted in humans around the world, and as many are underway for various metabolic, rheumatological, and neurological diseases, for example, to repair spinal cord injuries. Clinical research on the treatment of eye diseases with stem cells also remains very dynamic. An American team was thus able to produce from iPSCs an anatomically correct and functional human cornea. In 2019, a Japanese patient was able to benefit from a "sheet" of corneal cells, thus produced in the laboratory from iPSC cells.[1]

However, it is in cardiology that interest in stem cells is currently the most sustained, with the aim of functionally regenerating the diseased heart muscle. Patients who suffered a heart attack were treated by receiving heart cells derived from human stem cells, adsorbed on a fibrin patch. Other approaches involve directly administering the stem cells into the patient's heart in order to generate new muscle cells. The initial results of these studies are encouraging, with an improvement in both the cardiac function and physical condition of the patients thus treated. Moreover, at the stage of exploratory research, mini-human hearts are now produced in the laboratory from induced stem cells, which could eventually be used in transplantation to compensate for the deficit of available organs.

Although regenerative medicine is still at an experimental stage, the illegal and unregulated use of stem cells for therapeutic purposes has exploded in some countries over the past 10 years. For example, a trade in stem cells derived from umbilical cord blood has developed between the United States and Mexico. In China, unauthorized clinical studies have been conducted, and some hospitals offer medical tourism enthusiasts stem cell-based treatments whose effectiveness has not been proven. Several clinics in Florida and California have also offered treatments based on stem cells isolated from the adipose tissue or bone marrow of wealthy patients. This proliferation of commercial activities is worrying, as the origin, the production, and the modalities of use of stem cells are strictly regulated by the FDA, which to date has not authorized any stem cell treatment in humans.

To regulate research and prevent the marketing of unproven therapies, recommendations were issued as early as 2008 in the United States in order to avoid any uncontrolled use of stem cells derived from embryos. In 2016, the International Society for Stem Cell Research published new recommendations to enforce the regulations established by the FDA and ensure the origin as well as the quality of the cells used. This regulatory framework appears necessary today to eventually allow the medical exploitation of stem cells to regenerate all types of organs or tissues. This gigantic potential remains, however, to be realized.

[1] In France, the Vision Institute is evaluating in collaboration with the company I-Stem the local administration of stem cells to restore the sight of blind patients, this approach having shown encouraging initial results in rats.

High-tech Transplantations, Artificial Organs, and Intelligent Prosthetics

Since the first heart transplant performed by Professor Christiaan Barnard in 1967 in Cape Town, South Africa, enormous progress has been made in organ transplantation. Today, in addition to hearts, organs such as the kidney, lung, liver, pancreas, stomach, and intestine, as well as tissues such as the cornea, bone marrow, vein, artery, bone, cartilage, tendons, and ligaments are commonly transplanted. More sporadically, hand transplants, entire face transplants, and even the use of the first artificial organs have been undertaken successfully. The success rate of these transplants has significantly increased, thanks to surgical advances, but also because of the use of immunosuppressive drugs that prevent the rejection of the graft from the donor by the recipient's immune system.

However, in view of these needs, the shortage of organs available for transplantation remains a crucial challenge to overcome, and researchers are now turning to new technologies to remedy this. As mentioned earlier, xenotransplantation, the production of humanized organs in animals, and the use of mini-organs created in the laboratory from stem cells are among the avenues explored. Here, we will focus on two other particularly promising areas of research, namely 3D printing aiming to print biocompatible materials and biological tissues, as well as the development of medical devices and artificial organs implantable in the human body.

3D printing technology opens up new horizons in transplantation, thanks, on the one hand, to its relatively low cost and, on the other hand, to the very high precision of the printing. Guided by computer modeling from medical images, it allows for the creation of transplants perfectly adapted to the patient's anatomical characteristics. After transplantation, the printed biocompatible matrices are colonized by the patient's cells, promoting the reconstitution of an organ substitute. This technology is today increasingly used in orthopedic surgery to create artificial bones, as well as custom hip or knee prostheses.[2] Other applications of 3D printing include the production of biological tissues by depositing layers of organic materials and cells in order to reproduce the structure and composition of a natural tissue. For the first time in 2022, an American patient with a congenital malformation received an ear implant printed from a mix of her own cartilage cells and a hydrogel. At the experimental stage, several specialized biotechs are capable of printing prototypes of complex organs, such as miniature hearts, mini-kidneys, and liver fragments.[3] In the

[2] 3D printing is thus used by the company OsseoMatrix to produce a graft made from ceramic powder. This is gradually absorbed after colonization in a few months by the patient's bone cells. Japanese researchers use 3D printing to produce artificial bones from a mold made to the dimensions of the patient's bone to be replaced. This method could be applied to the hundreds of thousands of patients who, every year, are waiting for a bone graft worldwide. A Dutch medical team recently produced a fragment of a plastic skull with a 3D printer for a patient whose cranial bones were thickening to dangerously compress her brain.

[3] The printed ear was designed by the company 3DBio Therapeutics. Many companies have specialized in printing living tissues, such as Gorgé, OBL or Poietis. The mini-organs printed, a few cubic millimeters in size, can be preserved in the laboratory while remaining functional for several

printing of these small living organs, a remaining difficulty is to ensure their vascularization, that is, their irrigation by blood vessels to allow their oxygenation and their correct functioning over time.

In parallel to printed tissues, another high-tech advancement concerns the use of implants and prostheses to replace a deficient organ or a missing limb (see Box 4.1).

Box 4.1: Implants and Artificial Organs

For more than 60 years, different types of implants and medical devices have been commonly used for body repairs. In developed countries, one in five people over 65 currently benefits from an implant or a prosthesis. These include dental implants, *stents* to restore the blood flow in an obstructed vessel, intraocular lenses in case of cataracts, digital aids for the hearing impaired, *pacemakers* or valves to regulate heart rhythm disorders, hip or knee prostheses, and an insulin pump implanted under the skin for patients with diabetes. In the particular case of severe renal insufficiency, the filtration function of the kidney cannot yet be miniaturized in an artificial implantable device, so it is currently ensured by a dialysis machine outside the body.

From a futuristic perspective, technological advances aim to replace the entire organ with an intelligent artificial equivalent, taking advantage of the combined progress in biocompatible materials and flexible electronics. At different levels of development, work focuses on artificial versions of the pancreas, kidney (in the form of a portable dialysis system), lung, larynx, or even the eye [1]. The most advanced work in this field is that of the French company, Carmat, which, in early 2017, transplanted five patients with terminal heart failure with an artificial heart. Although these first transplanted patients all died after a few months, these results were encouraging, as they were obtained in patients condemned in the short term due to the advanced stage of their disease. At the end of 2020, Carmat's artificial heart received certification from European regulatory authorities to be used in patients with terminal heart failure while waiting for the transplantation of a real heart.

With the emergence of miniaturized electronics on supports compatible with the motility of living organisms, more and more "intelligent" medical devices can now be placed outside the body or implanted. This technology offers promising prospects for amputees by allowing a connectivity between the prosthesis and the nervous system of the residual tissue to provide the patient with better control of their prosthesis and a real sensory perception [2]. An example is the Myo-arm band, which forearm or hand amputees wear around their residual limb. This band, equipped with sensors, allows the operation of an artificial hand to grasp objects by

days in an optimized nutritional environment. The company 3D Bioprinting Solutions has printed a thyroid that proved functional after grafting to a mouse. This same company is now striving to print a functional kidney that could soon be transplanted into a human.

detecting the patient's muscle contractions when they mimic the desired action. Other development projects, such as connected cochlear implants to restore hearing and artificial retinas to improve vision, offer new hopes to people with severe hearing or visual deficits.[4]

These intelligent prostheses used in the health field foreshadow spectacular future human-machine hybridizations. A currently explored frontier is the interfacing of the human nervous system with electronics to allow computer control by thought. A first step in this direction was taken by Intel to assist the famous English physicist Stephen Hawking, who was suffering from amyotrophic lateral sclerosis (commonly called Charcot's or Lou Gehrig's disease), a disease that affects the motor neurons of the cerebral cortex and causes progressive muscle paralysis. This system allowed Hawking to compose letters or choose words on a computer by detecting the movements of his cheeks via a sensor placed in his glasses. A voice synthesizer then returned the selected words in the form of audible sentences. Current research is oriented toward the implantation of electrodes, placed directly into the brains of severely disabled people, in order to detect the electrical signals related to the movement of their lips, tongue, vocal box, or jaws. Using software, the speech intentions of the patients could then be transmitted to a voice synthesizer that would translate them into sounds.

In parallel, a neuroprosthesis was developed by the Polytechnic School of Lausanne to restore the ability to walk in macaques whose spinal cord had been injured. This neuroprosthesis, now being tested in humans, is a brain-machine interface that detects brain activity related to the intention to walk, then emits electrical stimuli to mobilize the walking muscles. Another approach to restoring motor skills involves using intelligent exoskeletons into which disabled people can slip to move. Quadriplegic patients thus receive cranial implants equipped with microelectrodes that detect their brain waves. These can then be interpreted by software to mobilize their limbs by thought, by controlling the movements of an exoskeleton.[5]

---

[4] The cochlear implants currently under development aim to restore hearing by establishing a connection between sensors placed in the failing ear and the patient's auditory nerve. Prototypes of artificial retinas under study are presented in the form of a silicon chip implanted in the patient's eye, which stimulates the retina so that it transmits to the brain electrical signals via the optic nerve. The most advanced projects for the development of artificial retinas concern the Argus II prostheses from the American Second Sight, Retina implant from the German AG, and the Iris II and Prima systems from the French Pixium Vision. These bionic retinas have already allowed patients blind from age-related macular degeneration or pigmentary retinopathies to recover part of their visual capacity.

[5] These technologies also arouse the interest of the military, who are developing prototypes of exoskeletons to allow soldiers to move over long distances or to carry heavy loads, such as HULC (*Human Universal Load Carrier*) or TALOS (*Tactical Assault Light Operator Suit*).

Nanomedicines, Nanoformulations, and Nanorobots

In 1959, Caltech researcher Richard Feynman proposed the crazy idea of building objects as thin as a sheet of paper by manipulating materials on an infinitely small scale. Thus, was born the concept of nanotechnologies, that is, technologies allowing the manipulation of matter on a scale ranging from the nanometer (10^{-9} m or one billionth of a meter) to the micron (10^{-6} m or one millionth of a meter).[6] Why should we be interested in the nanoworld populated by objects resulting from the assembly of a few atoms? Controlling the shape and size of the structures at the atomic scale allows obtaining objects with particularly interesting physical properties. For example, molecules such as fullerenes, composed of 60 carbon atoms assembled in the form of a nanoscale football, have proven to be remarkable superconductors. Other molecular structures based on carbon atoms, such as nanotubes or nanocones, have the particularity of producing extremely resistant materials.

Nanotechnologies rely not only on the ability of chemists to create original molecules by manipulating atoms but also on technologies such as tunnel microscopy, nanoscans, and electronic tweezers, which allow for the visualization and manipulation of atoms with precision. Note for the anecdote that the creation of an object the thickness of a sheet of paper by moving atoms one by one, as Richard Feynman had imagined, would take about 13,000 years! To speed up the process, scientists have therefore turned to methods based on the self-assembly of matter, inspired by living things.[7] The global market for nanotechnologies is currently estimated at USD 125 billion, with applications not only in materials and electronics, but also in chemistry and health.

The specific uses in the pharmaceutical field are multiple, ranging from drug formulation and vectorization systems to medical imaging agents and diagnostic tests, paving the way for a future nanomedicine.[8] Numerous nanodrugs are under development, but some are already on the market. They typically come in the form of very small particles made from lipids, nanoemulsions, or polymers, which contain the active ingredient. These nanoparticles stabilize this active ingredient and facilitate its entry into the cells. These properties have been exploited with the success that is known by Pfizer and Moderna companies to formulate their mRNA vaccines against COVID-19, using lipid nanoparticles. The nanoliposomes can also be decorated with receptors grafted onto their surface in order to precisely target

[6] The European Commission defines nanotechnologies as "natural, accidentally formed or manufactured nanomaterials, containing free particles or in the form of aggregates or agglomerates, of which at least 50% of the particles in the numerical size distribution have one or more external dimensions between 1 nm and 100 nm".

[7] In the living world, matter is shaped by parallel assemblies operating at different scales, between atoms, molecules, cells and tissues to produce predetermined shapes and functionalities, programmed in the DNA that constitutes the genetic heritage.

[8] In France, applications in nanomedicine are explored by companies such as Axialys (vectorization), BioAlliance (nanoparticulate drugs), Cytoo (cellular tests), Fluigent (microfluidics), Fluoptics (in vivo imaging), Nanobiotix (cancer radiotherapy), as well as by the laboratories from CEA-Leti and the Galien Institute (Université Paris-Saclay) in the field of nanomedicines.

certain cells or molecules. Nanotechnologies are therefore particularly useful for creating drugs specifically targeting diseased tissues while minimizing the side effects on healthy tissues. Several nanomedicines (Abraxane®, Daunoxone®, DepoCyt®, Doxil®, Myocet®, MM-398®) are now used as chemotherapies to treat certain cancers. Others have been authorized as treatments against infectious diseases (Ambisome®, Amphotec®) or pain (DepoDur®, Exparel®).[9]

Nanoparticles also allow for the improvement of the diagnosis of many diseases by precisely targeting imaging agents—for example, a contrast agent, a fluorochrome, or a radioelement—on tissues of interest. A nanoformulation can also increase the effectiveness of biotherapies based on recombinant proteins or monoclonal antibodies by avoiding the rejection or degradation of these medicinal molecules.[10] Conversely, other nanoparticles are developed to target immune cells in order to inhibit them in the case of autoimmune or inflammatory diseases, or alternatively, to activate them to induce a strong immune response during vaccination against infectious agents or cancer cells.

Beyond nanomedicines, the health field is interested in other applications in the form of medical devices based on nanorobots. In his futuristic book *Engines of Creation*, published in 1986, Eric Drexler imagined tiny robots capable of moving autonomously, manipulating atoms, and assembling other robots. In connection with this idea, a particularly interesting prospective research field aims to introduce specific functionalities into inanimate matter to make it "intelligent." Although this may seem like science fiction, the first steps in this direction have already been taken. Projects like the *Realizing Programmable Matter* from the American agency DARPA (*Defense Advanced Research Projects Agency*) are trying to create nanomaterials capable of self-assembly and self-repair without human intervention, but also reactive to external *stimuli*. Boston MIT researcher Skylab Tibias is working on using printing technology to obtain matter with programmable functional properties, an approach referred to as 4D printing to reflect a form of intelligence, thus integrated into this matter [3, 4].

Along the same lines, the Nobel Prize in Chemistry in 2016 rewarded work on molecular complexes moving in a controlled manner on frames based on metallic atoms, in response to light signals, electrical signals, or temperature changes.[11] These researchers have somehow created a "nanocar" with wheels made of fullerene molecules, allowing the nanovehicle to move on a metallic surface! An official competition between nanocars took place as early as 2017, with vehicles made up of a few hundred atoms "propelled" by electrical impulses on a track of gold atoms

---

[9] See two general reviews on nanomedicines available on the Mediachimie.org site: P. Couvreur. *Les nanomédicaments: une approche intelligente pour le traitement des maladies sévères*; E. Fattal. *Nanotechnologies pour la nanomedicine: questions sur la toxicité et aspects réglementaires.*

[10] Therapeutic antibodies used against cancers or inflammatory diseases often induce in the patient other antibodies directed against them, which can reduce their effectiveness. Nanoparticulate formulations reducing their ability to stimulate the immune system are therefore very interesting for preserving the effectiveness of these biotherapies, commonly used to treat patients for life.

[11] This Nobel Prize was jointly awarded to the Frenchman Jean-Pierre Sauvage, the British James Fraser Stoddart and the Dutchman Bernard Feringa.

100 nm long, which they had to cover in less than 36 h! As amusing as this first edition of the *NanoCar Race* may seem, the stakes here are very serious, perhaps foreshadowing future intelligent nanomedicines controllable externally by the therapist or the patient to deliver the active principle at the right place and at the right time. In parallel, another small robot in the form of a fluid structure composed of magnetic nanoparticles has been developed by other researchers. Controllable by an external magnet, this robot could eventually transport a drug in the human body. These molecular machines may prefigure the intelligent medical nanodevices that, in the future, will be injected into the bodies of patients to deliver a targeted drug, destroy blood clots or cancer cells, or even eliminate infectious agents.

A Synthetic Biology with No Limit

Synthetic biology aims to design and produce molecules or biological organisms with useful properties, particularly in the health field. Its ambition is not only to modify existing biological substrates but also to create entirely new ones to obtain revolutionary therapies. To this end, this field of research does not rule out any possibility of manipulating the functional characteristics of cells and molecules, far beyond a simple exploitation of their natural properties.

Synthetic biology is particularly interested in technologies that can synthesize increasingly long strands of DNA or RNA in order to create modified or artificial genes and chromosomes. Entrepreneur Craig Venter and his team—the same ones who contributed to sequencing the human genome—were the first to synthesize a simple natural genome in 2010, that of a bacterium of the genus *Chlamydia*. In 2014, a yeast chromosome containing 270,000 nucleotide pairs was in turn entirely synthesized in the laboratory. The genetic material thus produced is still very simple compared to the human genome, the latter comprising nearly 12,000 times the number of nucleotides contained in a yeast! The synthesis of a human genome remains to this day a monumental project, only conceivable through a global public–private consortium, with a pilot project, named *Human Genome Project-Write*, already initiated in 2016 for this purpose.[12] The cost of DNA sequencing has dropped significantly (by 8 logarithms in base 10) since the 2000s, but the cost of DNA synthesis (which has only dropped by 2 to 3 logs) remains prohibitive in view of the challenge of synthesizing the 3 billion base pairs contained in a human genome. Another technical difficulty lies in the insertion of such a large quantity of DNA in a cell so that it can be read and produce proteins.

The synthesis of RNA strands is particularly interesting for creating new drugs, as demonstrated by RNA vaccines against COVID-19. The RNAs usable as active ingredients in this application are small in size and can therefore be easily produced

[12] The term "writing" refers here to the synthesis of DNA, in mirror to sequencing which consists in "reading" the DNA. This pilot project was initiated at a reduced cost (about 3 billion US dollars!), in order to synthesize in a first-time human chromosome fragments and then check their functionality.

with current technologies. Their sequence can be modified as needed by changing one or more nucleotides compared to the natural sequence, and it is possible to create RNAs coding for completely new proteins. This versatility in RNA synthesis, demonstrated with anti-COVID-19 vaccines, allows us to consider other applications in vaccinology, for example, to protect against the many variants of influenza, AIDS, or hepatitis C viruses. Moreover, these RNA drugs are now considered for vaccinating patients with cancer against antigens specifically carried by their tumor, with preliminary results encouraging in patients with pancreatic cancer, a particularly aggressive cancer for which there is no satisfactory treatment.[13]

Beyond its considerable promise, synthetic biology also raises questions about the potential risks associated with the creation of artificial organisms with undesirable properties. Given the deliberate transgression of known natural boundaries, the risk is not only theoretical. A team from the Scripps Research Institute in California reported in 2017 the synthesis of artificial nucleotides called X and Y, replicable by the cellular machinery in the same way as natural nucleotides, after insertion into a bacterium. By thus extending the alphabet of life, synthetic biology has opened the way to the creation and reprogramming of all kinds of natural, artificial, or hybrid life forms.[14] In a completely different application, research conducted at the University of Wisconsin–Madison has allowed researchers to recreate in the laboratory a flu virus particularly dangerous for humans. This virus indeed has 97% homology in its genomic sequence with the one that caused several tens of millions of deaths during the Spanish flu pandemic in 1918.[15] These studies aimed to better understand the mechanisms of transmission and virulence of the virus to improve treatments. However, the scientific community has been concerned about the risk of accidentally recreating a highly transmissible pathogen to humans in case of a breach of secure containment measures in the laboratory.

Given the nature of such work, a challenge is therefore to control not only the research conducted by experienced scientists in accredited laboratories but also the experiments carried out by the *biohackers* who indulge in biotechnologies in an

[13] Rojas et al. [5]. In this study, patients were treated with synthetic RNAs corresponding to antigens carried by their own tumor. These personalized synthetic vaccines were combined with chemotherapy and an immune checkpoint inhibitor. Half of the patients developed immune responses based on T lymphocytes capable of killing tumor cells. These vaccine responders benefited from a longer survival than that of non-responders. In parallel, Moderna announced in December 2023 that its RNA vaccine against melanoma prevented a recurrence after chemotherapy treatment in half of the patients.

[14] Zhang et al. [6]. The natural nucleotides that make up DNA are four in number, namely adenine, cytosine, guanine, and thymine, abbreviated by their initials A, C, G, T. The different combinations of these nucleotides with each other allow to code for 20 natural amino acids that make up the proteins of all known living organisms to date. With the creation of artificial nucleotides X and Y, replicable by living organisms, synthetic biology makes conceivable the extension of this natural genetic code from 4 to 6 letters. If, today, these artificial nucleotides do not allow to code for amino acids and therefore proteins, a first step has nevertheless been taken which allows to envisage future living organisms integrating totally new synthetic molecules…

[15] Kawaoka et al. [7]. This laboratory-produced virus contains genetic material from avian virus that makes it highly transmissible to humans.

unregulated manner.[16] In 2014, a group of international scientific experts was convened by the European Commission to assess the specific risks posed by synthetic biology. This committee concluded that existing controls needed to be adapted to ensure the safety of research in this field. Beyond the usual difficulties in assessing the risks associated with any new technology, synthetic biology raises the specific question of comparators, that is, known products that can be used as a reference to assess risks. In this field, the aim is to produce molecules or organisms radically different from anything that nature or human intelligence has designed so far. A recurring issue will be evaluating the products resulting from an innovation whose "*raison d'être*" is to operate in *terra incognita.*

References

1. Raguin T, et al. Artificial organs. Med Sci. 2017;33:66.
2. Raspopovic S. Advancing limb neural prosthesis. Science. 2020;370:290.
3. Drexler E. Engines of Creation: the coming era of nanotechnology. New York: Doubleday; 1986.
4. Rizza G. Impression 4D: Les matériaux intelligents du futur. Polytechnique-insights.com, February 2022.
5. Rojas L, et al. Personalized RNA neoantigen vaccines stimulate T cells in pancreatic cancer. Nature. 2023;618:144.
6. Zhang Y, et al. A semisynthetic organism engineered for the stable expansion of the genetic alphabet. Proc Natl Acad Sci USA. 2017;114:1317.
7. Kawaoka Y, et al. A highly pathogenic avian H7N9 influenza virus isolated from a human is lethal in some ferrets infected via respiratory droplets. Cell Host Microbe. 2017;22:615.

[16] It is estimated that tens of thousands of followers of the movement *do-it yourself* and *biohackers* around the world use biotechnologies in their garages, out of any control.

Part II

The Contributions of Artificial Intelligence to Medicine

5 New Momentum: Digital Health

Digital Transformation and Digital Medicine

Digital medicine, or e-health, includes all health-related services that use technologies such as the Internet, smartphone applications, or connected objects. Developed countries have implemented proactive policies to accelerate their digital transformation in strategic sectors, such as health. In France, public funding in the order of billions of euros is dedicated to improving the collection and use of health data, notably through the creation of a gigantic, centralized *Health data hub*.[1] Digital technologies and the improvement of IT infrastructures are indeed identified as essential levers to facilitate the capture, sharing, reuse, and storage of data for health.

Digital medicine relies in particular on connected objects and data interpretation software. The wellness and *fitness* sectors were the first to resort to sensors, bracelets, watches, and connected clothing to continuously measure blood pressure or body temperature. These objects also provide environmental data such as exposure to light and noise, and they can even inform about the subject's gait, this last parameter allowing the early detection of a muscular or neurological disease.[2] Beyond that, doctors now use decision algorithms to interpret health data in order to establish their diagnosis and determine the appropriate treatment. Pharmacists use specific software to identify drug incompatibilities or dosage errors in prescriptions.[3] In the United States, the FDA has thus approved several dozen software programs for

[1] The study report coordinated by Deputy Cédric Villani emphasized in 2018 the need to establish structures for collecting and sharing data. Article 47 of the French health system modernization law provides for the creation of a national system gathering health data from Health Insurance, local authorities and complementary insurances. The French Social Security system is also a very valuable source of data on the evolution of diseases and the responses to treatments.

[2] All data collected by these connected objects can be compiled on a smartphone or centralized on a secure server, to be made available to health professionals.

[3] The level of evidence required by health agencies regarding the reliability of these intelligent digital medical devices requires clinical studies whose results are included in the certification file.

P. Moingeon, *Intelligent Drugs: How AI is Transforming Healthcare*,
https://doi.org/10.1007/978-3-031-91668-7_5

data interpretation for therapeutic or diagnostic purposes, granting a status of *Clinical Decision Support*. Other intelligent devices, like the "bionic" artificial pancreas, have also been authorized to automatically regulate the glucose level measured in patients with diabetes by controlling the dose of insulin injected using a mini-pump.[4]

Intelligent digital devices are useful for improving adherence to medical treatments, that is, to help patients take their medications as prescribed by the doctor. Besides the fact that poorly followed treatments can lose effectiveness, let's remember that non-adherence in taking treatments causes about USD 100 billion per year in avoidable health costs worldwide! "Intelligent" tablets, including the Helios tablet from Futura Sciences, incorporate tiny chips containing the list of prescribed medications as well as their dosage. A sensor on the abdomen detects the intake of the tablet by the patient, thus confirming its ingestion to the doctor.[5] In 2017, the FDA approved the marketing of these connected pills for patients suffering from schizophrenia, bipolar disorders, and chronic diseases like high blood pressure, heart failure, or diabetes. These intelligent tablets prove particularly suitable for elderly patients taking several medications, as half of them do not take their treatment correctly.

Telemedicine is another application of digital technologies that is gaining in popularity. This recent practice allows complete remote care, from the appointment to the consultation, up to the prescription of care and follow-up. From the patients' point of view, telemedicine avoids going to the doctor, an advantage in case of geographical constraints or particular situations, like the COVID-19 pandemic. Digital technologies are also used by the pharmaceutical industry to carry out more and more decentralized clinical studies in order to evaluate the effectiveness of new drugs. In this approach, the number of hospital visits is significantly reduced, as patients are monitored remotely thanks to connected objects that collect their electronic health data.[6]

Another aspect of digital health is the care of patients by intelligent machines, thanks to voice interfaces. Voice assistants such as Siri, Alexa, or Google Home are frequently used to answer simple everyday life questions. But some of these devices

[4] Connected health tools are particularly useful for patients with diabetes. This chronic disease, which accounts for 10% of health expenditures in developed countries, indeed requires very regular monitoring of blood glucose levels. The company Medtronic has developed a sensor implanted under the skin that measures glucose levels in real time and controls a mini insulin pump. The company Diabeloop is also developing an artificial pancreas called DBLG1. The measurement of glucose to adjust the administration of insulin can also be done using sensors or corneal lenses connected to smartphones.

[5] A similar intelligent pill technology was developed in parallel by the Japanese laboratory Otsuka in collaboration with the company Proteus.

[6] Telemedicine also allows for the remote training of health professionals, as well as tele-expertise when caregivers need the opinion of colleagues at a distance. Augmented reality has also made its way into operating rooms. Using Microsoft's HoloLens glasses, surgeons can now operate on a patient while simultaneously visualizing a 3-dimensional hologram created from medical images to guide their movements with extreme precision.

also have interesting applications in health. For example, Amazon's Alexa software can diagnose certain diseases, such as an allergy, a cold, or even a suspicion of COVID-19, by analyzing the voice, breathing, or cough of the patient. It can also remind patients to take their medications according to the doctor's recommendations. On a large scale, the British company Babylon Health has been collaborating with the National Health Service (NHS) since 2017 to offer medical consultations by videoconference to its millions of users. In these interactions, a conversational robot (*chatbot*) analyzes the symptoms described by the patient over the phone. The software uses semantic recognition to interpret the patient's words, identify keywords, make a probable diagnosis, and suggest to the doctor an appropriate prescription of medications. With ChatGPT and, more generally, the new forms of generative AI based on very large language models (*LLMs*), chatbots capable of conducting a real autonomous conversation with the patient will be increasingly used in disease screening. The prospects of the global digital health market are estimated in the short term at USD 300 billion per year, which explains the interest shown by the giants of the Net technologies (GAFAMs and BATHX) in the development of digital tools in health, as we will discuss later.[7]

Most likely, all these digital tools will be endorsed by the patients themselves, allowing them to proactively manage their health. However, for the full development of digital medicine, the acceptability by regulatory authorities of the reliability and level of evidence provided by the collection and analysis of health data with these new tools will be very important. This recognition will also be crucial economically to allow for the coverage of this connected medicine by health systems.[8] Such a favorable evolution is anticipated in the short term, as it will be demonstrated that digital technologies improve the efficiency of care while reducing health costs.

The Intelligence of Machines

While digital technologies allow for the efficient collection and transmission of health data, their analysis to extract useful information is truly enabled by AI. In simple terms, AI is a set of theories, methods, and tools aimed at developing intelligent machines capable of reproducing certain dimensions of human intelligence, thanks to a convergence of technologies. Historically, the concept of an intelligent machine was theorized by several mathematicians in the middle of the twentieth century. Among them, the American–Hungarian John von Neumann analogously depicted the human brain as a machine capable of conceiving something more complex than itself. Another important actor was the American Norbert Wiener, founder of cybernetics, a scientific discipline devoted to the mechanisms of communication

[7] GAFAMs is the acronym that brings together the American companies Google, Apple, Facebook (now Meta), Amazon and Microsoft. BATHX refers to the Chinese digital giants Baidu, Alibaba, Tencent, Huawei and Xiaomi.

[8] In France, the Diabeo smartphone application allowing diabetic patients to monitor their blood sugar levels was reimbursed by social security in 2016.

and regulation used by living beings. However, it was the English mathematician Alan Turing who most explicitly formulated, in a famous article published in the journal *Mind* in 1950, this prescient hypothesis: sophisticated machines will one day be able to manifest certain forms of intelligence [1].

A definition of AI, proposed by Nils Nilsson, is that *artificial intelligence consists of making machines intelligent, and intelligence is that quality that allows an entity to function appropriately, with a perception of its environment* [2]. This definition has the advantage of considering that machines can perceive the surrounding world and act accordingly. We can add that intelligence, whether human or artificial, implies not only an ability to analyze but also to learn. In summary, AI aims to create "intelligent" machines that can perceive, analyze, act, learn, and, since the appearance of ChatGPT 3.5 in November 2022, communicate expressively (Table 5.1).

In practice, AI relies on all sources of data, including sensors, cameras, and connected devices, which collect real-time data on the environment (perception). These data are interpreted by computers with constantly increasing computing power, which produce models of complex problems (analysis). These models help humans make decisions and act appropriately, either by themselves or through machines, such as robots. Intelligent machines have recently become capable of learning, which allows them to continuously improve their predictive models.

There are several types of machine learning, supervised or unsupervised, depending on whether the data are previously annotated by humans to be exploited by the machine. We also discuss deep learning to evoke the training of intelligent machines in the form of artificial neural networks to develop predictive algorithms, using large amounts of data covering, for example, existing human knowledge on a given subject. The word algorithm, which is derived from the name of the Persian mathematician Al-Khwârizmî (nineteenth century), now refers to a series of instructions and mathematical operations allowing the solution of a type of problem. Deep learning has been made possible thanks to the work of Yann Le Cun and colleagues on the use of artificial neural networks inspired by the functioning of the visual cortex of primates in order to interpret images [3, 4].

More generally, the idea of an "intelligent" machine is based on the analogy between the functioning of computers and that of the primate brain. Many intelligent machines use networks of small computing units (as "neurons"), assembled in parallel layers to mimic the synaptic connections of the human brain. Each layer contains hundreds of artificial neurons, and these networks can process information (in the form of binary language, 0 or 1) much faster than their biological equivalents, which explains their high computing capacity. They can thus analyze huge amounts of data and be trained to identify and classify images with remarkable efficiency.[9]

[9] In this application, the neurons of the first layer of the network receive input signals that they transmit or not, depending on predefined thresholds, to the neurons of the next layer in the form of output signals. These signals propagate from layer to layer, gradually extracting the necessary information to categorize the images.

Table 5.1 Features of human intelligence reproduced by machines

Features	Human being	Intelligent machine
Perception	Perception of the environment (images, sounds, smells, tastes, textures) thanks to the sensory organs and the peripheral and central nervous systems	Sensors, cameras, microphones, and connected objects allow for the collection and transmission in real time of data on the environment (images, sounds, textures, analytical parameters)
Analysis	Integration and analysis by the central nervous system of the information provided by the sensory organs	Analysis of massive and diverse data thanks to computing power, allowing the establishment of a model, that is to say, a representation of physical reality. These models, which can be predictive, are useful to humans for making decisions and guiding their actions
Action	Reflex or voluntary motor action, manifesting an intention or an impulse, involving nerve endings and muscles (with release of neurotransmitters at the neuromuscular junction) Human actions can be delegated to automata or robots	Execution by programmed or autonomous machines and robots of repetitive, painful, ultra-precise, or dangerous tasks, potentially in hostile environments or inaccessible to humans
Learning	Knowledge is acquired through observation, education, experience, and memory	Multiple modalities of machine learning (also called automatic learning), including supervised or unsupervised learning and deep or reinforced learning, are based on the integration and analysis of data to train and then update algorithms, that is, the mathematical operations that underlie predictive models
Expressive communication	Speech and writing involving the mastery and semantic understanding of language	Analysis and understanding of written and spoken human language (natural language processing, natural language understanding), and reproduction of this language by voice synthesis. These functionalities have significantly developed with the emergence of conversational agents like ChatGPT in late 2022. This form of generative AI, based on large language models, now allows intelligent machines to communicate with humans autonomously, beyond the simple programming of responses to a limited list of questions

Beyond a definition of AI as a convergence of technologies that reproduces certain properties of human intelligence, this question arises: what is it for? The essential functionality provided by AI consists of the analysis of data in very large quantities, but also very diverse. Thanks to AI and machine learning, it has become possible to integrate this data, whether it is structured (i.e., formatted in a database to facilitate computer exploitation) or unstructured. Importantly, the latter, which were hitherto unexploitable prior to the emergence of AI, represent up to 90% of the data produced by humanity. As we have seen, advances in molecular profiling technologies and medical imaging generate significant amounts of multimodal data on the patient. Together, digital technologies and AI now offer considerably increased possibilities for capturing, sharing, integrating, and analyzing this data.

This new opportunity allows for many applications in the field of health, particularly to accelerate the design and development of innovative drugs for the benefit of patients. The revolution now underway, as we will see, was only made possible very recently, when AI reached maturity.

Why Will AI Transform Health?

Since its birth in the middle of the twentieth century, AI has experienced—as predicted by Amara's law—periods of enthusiasm, but also "winters" caused by obstacles that have long prevented it from fulfilling its promises. For about a decade, it has generated exponential interest in all fields of activity, especially in health, where the market for AI applications could reach USD 200 billion by 2030, up from just USD 8 billion in 2020!

The maturity of AI has been made possible thanks to three major advancements. First, progress in computational sciences has allowed the development of increasingly powerful processors, significantly increasing the computing capacity. Then, the development of very efficient machine learning methods, particularly deep learning, has been used to train artificial neural networks with large amounts of data to obtain high-performance predictive algorithms. Finally, the predicted golden age for AI is only possible thanks to a third factor: the availability of abundant data. These data are currently produced by humanity on the scale of zettabytes (i.e., 10^{21} bytes) per year, with an annual growth of 40% observed over the last decade![10] These data are generated thanks to audiovisual technologies, multimedia, the Internet, and connected objects that continuously provide images, texts, sounds, semantic content, and analytical data. The exploitation of these data is also greatly facilitated not only by advances in their capture but also by their curation, sharing, and large-scale storage, notably thanks to digital technologies, including cloud computing.[11]

A major contribution of AI is not only to be able to "ingest" this massive data, whatever its form, but also to capture its value by producing models usable by humans to assist them in their decisions and actions. A model constitutes a simplified representation of a problem or a physical phenomenon in the form of a system of components and their interactions. The very first models created by humans were obviously constructed without the aid of computers. For example, a model of a theoretical animal was used at the end of the nineteenth century by the French zoologist

[10] Eberendu [5]. In comparison, it is estimated that the human brain is capable of storing about one petabyte (or 10^{15} bytes) of data.

[11] Curation involves the selection and editing of data to improve its quality.

Paul Bert to teach students the coordinated functioning of organs in the animal kingdom. The objective of Paul Bert's model was not to faithfully reproduce an existing animal but rather to describe and explain in general terms the functioning of the main organs that constitute an animal. Thanks to AI, extremely powerful and scalable models of complex issues can now be envisaged. Depending on the level of information and knowledge they allow to be extracted from raw data, four types of models are distinguished. The simplest is that of a description of the system's components. Beyond that, a model can have diagnostic value, helping to understand the nature of this system. We recognize here two functionalities achieved by Bert's model. At a more informative level, the models produced by AI allow predictions to be made, for example, on the evolution of the system if one of its components is disturbed. This predictive modeling can even go as far as a prescriptive analysis, suggesting to humans some modes of action in the real world while anticipating the consequences. In this book, we will be particularly interested in predictive and prescriptive AI-based models used to, on the one hand, represent the specificities of the patient and, on the other hand, predict the properties of multiple drug candidates in order to decide accordingly which drug will be most appropriate to treat this patient.

The contribution of AI in the predictive and prescriptive exploitation of data opens a wide range of applications in all sectors of human activity. These applications are related to weak AI, which relies on intelligent machines designed to efficiently execute specific tasks for which they have been programmed. This weak AI is distinguished from strong AI, also called general intelligence or superintelligence, which arouses the interest of some researchers and could, in an uncertain future, lead to the emergence of autonomous machines endowed with a capacity to perform any intellectual task a human can, with their own intentions, even completely emancipating themselves from any human control.[12]

The weak AI that constitutes the state of the art today has begun to transform our daily lives, with applications as varied as image analysis, psychological profiling of customers to provide personalized services and products, the development of autonomous vehicles, robot control, and the design of ultra-connected smart cities. AI allows real-time counting of objects or vehicles, analysis and regulation of flows, predictive maintenance of tools, quality control of products, and production processes. It is applied to facial recognition, video surveillance, biometric controls at borders, and anti-terrorist or anti-criminal fights. AI applications are now being deployed as part of the digital transformation of manufacturing industries, hospitals, and administrations in order to improve data sharing and exploitation and thereby the coordination of activities and alignment of resources in complex organizations. A particular field in considerable expansion concerns the analysis and

[12] Many experts doubt the possibility of the emergence of strong AI. Some, however, believe it has a 90% chance of appearing by 2075 (see N. Bostrom, *Superintelligence*, Oxford University Press, 2014). The recent emergence of large language models, like ChatGPT, could be a first step towards strong AI. Various scenarios of the emergence of strong AI, with speculations about its interactions more or less friendly towards humans, have been envisaged by Ted Mark, a physicist at MIT in Boston, in his book *Life 3.0*, Penguin books, 2017.

understanding by computers of natural language (NLP, or natural language processing, and NLU, or natural language understanding), combined with voice synthesis. It is now possible to perform, thanks to AI, ultra-fast semantic analysis of large amounts of written or spoken texts.

In this regard, at the end of 2022, a new form of AI appeared to the general public with ChatGPT, based on large language models. LLMs use specific artificial neural networks, known as *transformers*. These AI solutions, specialized in understanding and generating human language, are trained on billions of words from books, articles, and websites. When a sentence or a question is presented to them, they predict the following words (or, more precisely, fragments called *tokens*) thanks to an astonishing probabilistic prediction capacity acquired by learning from huge amounts of text. GPT (which stands for *Generative Pre-trained Transformer*) is a famous example, capable of autonomously answering questions posed by humans. Indeed, generative AI is so named because, from the data it has been fed, it creates new texts, images, music, or videos in response to user requests. It offers remarkable potentialities by automating tasks such as writing and translating texts, generating code, synthesizing complex information, providing educational assistance, and answering everyday questions.[13]

With these advances, the applications of AI are numerous in health. AI radically transforms medical diagnosis and screening by allowing an interpretation of biological or imaging results and a detailed analysis of patients' medical records. Artificial neural networks are particularly effective for analyzing and classifying images, with multiple medical uses. AI is thus able to detect early signs of diseases from images, or even predict them, thereby greatly improving the chances of successful treatments. It contributes to the improvement of hospital management and health systems and promotes better patient care. By exploiting massive and varied databases, AI transforms drug research, allowing a better understanding of disease mechanisms and the design of more personalized, more effective, and safer drugs. However, this abundance of concrete applications currently being explored is only the very beginning of the incredible evolution that will occur in health in the relatively short term. The potential in the biomedical field is all the greater as AI is set to progress considerably in each of the technologies that compose it.

As an example, a particularly active field of research remains self-learning, with different learning methods—supervised, unsupervised, deep, and reinforced (Table 5.1). We have pointed out that supervised learning relies on the use of data labeled by humans to develop algorithms. In an unsupervised approach, no rule is provided to the machine that categorizes the data without a priori. Deep learning, for example, in the form of training artificial neural networks with large amounts of data, has the interest of creating forms of AI progressively capable of learning by themselves, without being programmed by humans. Reinforced learning also allows the machine to continuously learn by itself in response to a reward received for its

[13] See Grinbaum [6]. This essay questions the philosophical and societal implications of these new machines capable of having real conversations with humans, while being unable to think or understand what they "say".

correct answers. This learning method was used to train the AlphaGo software, which in 2016 beat the world Go champion, Lee Sedol. This transition toward self-learning machines is not without consequence; the acquisition of greater autonomy by machines leads to a progressive decrease in their control by humans.

Equally spectacular advances are taking place, which concern the computing power of intelligent machines, allowing the ever faster analysis of gigantic amounts of data. As these lines are written, the most powerful computer in the world is the Fugaku 415-PFLOPs supercomputer, set up in Japan in 2021, with a computing power of 442 petaflops (*Floating Point Operations Per Second*), that is, several hundred million billion calculations per second![14] This computer was installed at the Riken Institute in Tokyo, notably to extend the capabilities of designing new chemical molecules, an activity that requires great computing power. This could well be further increased by using chips based on DNA or carbon nanotubes, allowing for the storage and analysis of more information. If these advances are realized, the increase in computational power will far exceed the limits predicted by Moore's law.[15]

At the same time, quantum computing is generating a lot of interest in the race for computer performance. This developing technology relies on the quantum properties of matter, such as entanglement and superposition, to increase the data processing power. Unlike traditional computers, which process binary data (with values of 0 or 1), quantum computers analyze data at the scale of *qubits*, the smallest known units of information storage to date.[16] Quantum computing offers the promise of manipulating almost unlimited amounts of data, a feature that is particularly interesting in the world of medicine. Companies—like the French company Qbit Pharmaceuticals—are already exploring the application of this technology to the design of novel drug molecules. Increased computing power will also be essential for a futuristic application that we will revisit, which aims to create digital avatars of each individual in order to test drugs—virtual or real—by computer!

[14] This computer developed by the company Fujitsu uses processors based on chips with a very good energy efficiency. The Summit and Sierra supercomputers designed by IBM, respectively 2nd and 3rd most powerful in the world, develop a computing power of about 149 and 95 petaflops, respectively. In comparison, the first supercomputer *Blue Gene*, created in 2005 by IBM, was at the time capable of processing 360 teraflops. The suffixes peta and tera correspond respectively to the numbers 10^{15} and 10^{12}; that is to say that the latest generation supercomputers have, in less than 20 years, acquired a computing power more than 1000 times greater than *Blue Gene*!

[15] Service [7]. Moore's law, stated by Gordon Moore, one of the founders of Intel in 1965, correctly predicted that the number of transistors on an electronic chip—and thereby their power—would double every 18 months. This law has reached a physical limit related to current silicon supports; however, the use of new storage supports could re-energize the race forward. American military research programs, such as *the Electronic Resurgence Initiative* of the American DARPA agency, aim to improve the efficiency of chips using carbon nanotubes, capable of activating and deactivating more quickly than current silicon transistors.

[16] The first quantum processor was developed by Yale University in 2009. It consisted of two qubits each composed of a billion aluminum atoms adsorbed on a superconducting matrix. IBM unveiled at the Consumer Electronics Show in Las Vegas in 2019 the first commercial quantum computer called System Q.

References

1. Turing A. Computing machinery and intelligence. Mind. 1950;59:433.
2. Nilsson N. The quest for artificial intelligence: a history of ideas and achievements. Cambridge: Cambridge University Press; 2010.
3. Le Cun Y, Bengio Y, Hinton G. Deep learning. Nature. 2015;521:436.
4. Le Cun Y. Quand la machine apprend. La revolution des neurones artificiels et de l'apprentissage profond. Paris: Odile Jacob; 2019.
5. Eberendu AC. Unstructured data: an overview of the data of big data. Int J Comput Trends Technol. 2016;38:46.
6. Grinbaum A. Machine words. Paris: Humensciences; 2023.
7. Service R. Chipmakers look past Moore law and silicon. Science. 2018;361:321.

6 The AI-Augmented Patient

Deciphering the Human Singularity

Recent scientific advances have taught us that each individual is unique. As we have seen, genome sequencing, epigenetic analyses, and characterization of microbiota allow us to highlight particularities of each individual at the molecular level, linked not only to their biological heritage but also to their relationship with the environment and their life experience.[1]

Knowledge of our singularity is possible in the first place at the biological level, notably through the exploitation of genetic data. High-throughput DNA and RNA sequencing technologies now allow the investigation of genetic polymorphisms at the population level. Comparative studies of genomic sequences of many individuals have revealed differences, in the form of mutations or point variations in DNA sequences, specific to each individual. SNPs (*Single Nucleotide Polymorphisms*) mentioned earlier constitute minor modifications of the genome, but they can have important functional consequences, such as susceptibility or, on the contrary, resistance to a disease. In order to better understand the nature and the scope of these variations within our species, significant resources are currently devoted to the automated sequencing of the genomes of millions of individuals in different geographical regions, whether they are healthy or suffering from various diseases. The American company Illumina is a major player in this research, thanks to its devices capable of sequencing a human genome in a few hours. Applied on an industrial

[1] Even true homozygous twins, that is, those from the same fertilized egg and having an identical genetic heritage, do not express exactly the same traits due to their distinct lifestyles. This would also be true if an individual was cloned: the original subject and its clone would have a very similar physical appearance, but their eating habits, their stress level, their exposure to pollution would be different. These differences would be biologically translated by epigenetic modifications of their DNA and by distinct microbiota.

P. Moingeon, *Intelligent Drugs: How AI is Transforming Healthcare*,
https://doi.org/10.1007/978-3-031-91668-7_6

scale, the HiSeq X technology, developed by Illumina, now allows the sequencing of 20,000 genomes per year, at a unit cost of about USD 1000 per genome.[2]

A comparative analysis of genome sequencing data is underway in laboratories around the world, thanks to collaborative projects such as ENCODE (*Encyclopedia of DNA elements*) and the *Human Variome Project*. These initiatives aim to establish a catalog of human genetic variations. In parallel, international research is interested in the second genome, the microbiome. Since 2019, a considerable effort has been undertaken to sequence millions of microbiomes from different parts of the body, with the aim of creating a reference map for the human species. This research also aims to understand the role of the microbiome in the predisposition to various diseases and to design new drugs targeting the microbiota.[3] By combining this knowledge, we will be able, in the near future, to better understand the nature and extent of human biological variability, the interactions between genes and the environment, as well as the relationship between these polymorphisms and many diseases.

The biological characterization data obtained through complete genome sequencing and multi-omic analysis of blood or tissues allow us to document all biological processes, metabolisms, and hormonal systems. In addition, they allow us to measure specific organ parameters that reflect their proper functioning or aging. These data can be complemented by other quantitative and qualitative information about the patients' relationship with their environment, such as their diet, physical exercise practice, alcohol and tobacco consumption, and any other potential addictions. Profiling will also integrate the characterization of their intestinal, respiratory, genital, and skin microbiota, as well as their exposome, that is, their exposure profile to pollutants, allergens, toxic products, and infectious agents, measured in their daily environment.

In addition to these highly sophisticated biological typings, high-resolution medical imaging technologies are also very interesting for documenting the specifics of each individual patient's disease. Digital radiology, computed tomography (CT scan), positron emission tomography, magnetic resonance imaging, and echography using ultrasound are different methods that allow detailed observation of the structure and functioning of organs in a non-invasive way.[4] These different medical

---

[2] Such devices (which cost about one $ million US each) also make it possible to consider the sequencing of millions of genomes, for example from cancer cells, plants, animals and bacterial ecosystems. China, particularly active in this field, has two specialized companies, BGI and Novogen, which together account for about 30% of the world's DNA sequencing power.

[3] Let's remember that the word microbiota describes the set of bacteria, viruses, and fungi that colonize our body, while the microbiome encompasses the genetic material associated with these microorganisms. The consortium *Million Microbiome of Humans Project* brings together the BGI Research Institute and the Shanghai National Clinical Research Center for Metabolic Diseases in China, the Karolinska Institute in Sweden, the University of Copenhagen in Denmark, and the National Institute for Agricultural Research (INRA) in France.

[4] X-ray based radiography provides two-dimensional snapshots of a tissue or organ, while the scanner uses rotating X-rays to create cross-sectional images and reconstruct 3D images. Echography analyzes the ultrasound absorbed or reflected by tissues. Magnetic resonance imaging (MRI) relies

imaging techniques have made considerable progress in recent years. Beyond better image resolution, interpretation software and advances in virtual reality allow the integration of several images to create an accurate three-dimensional representation of organs, lesions, and tumors.

Medical imaging has become a privileged field of application for AI in health. Indeed, artificial neural networks are particularly effective in image analysis, allowing the automated detection of well-defined pathological profiles. In 2017, Stanford University confirmed in the journal *Nature* that algorithms trained from millions of medical images could detect skin cancers—specifically melanomas—with the same reliability as seasoned dermatologists. With the progress of computer vision, this level of performance, equivalent to that of the best human experts, is now extended to all types of medical images [1, 2]. This medical imaging enhanced by AI is already improving early disease diagnosis and facilitating targeted therapeutic and surgical interventions. A significant advantage of the intelligent machine is that it can perform automated image analysis at a very high speed after programming. It is estimated that the machine can analyze up to 250 million medical images per day for a total cost of USD 1000! However, the limitation is that AI only detects the anomalies for which it has been programmed, unlike human experts trained to detect all types of alterations. Therefore, the responsibility for diagnosis based on AI-assisted medical image analysis will remain, for a few more years, a prerogative of human experts.

The exploitation of all these molecular profiling and medical imaging data is now possible, thanks to AI, to decipher the characteristics of each human being with an unprecedented level of detail. As we will see, this knowledge will allow, in the medium term, the prediction of the evolution of the health of each individual, sick or healthy, from birth to death.

The Patient of the Future, Manager of His Health

As we move further into the twenty-first century, patients will be better taken care of not only by this precision medicine but also by themselves. They will become central actors in their own health. Perfectly informed of their weaknesses and specific risks, they will be fully aware that they can shape their health through their lifestyle. When affected by a chronic disease with age, patients will want to continue living normally. These legitimate expectations will profoundly change their relationship with health professionals, who will have to deal with patients eager to participate in all health decisions concerning them.

This patient of the future, engaged at the center of the care network as a manager of his health, already exists; his name is "Larry the Transparent." This is the

on electromagnetic waves to provide images of organs by measuring the signals emitted by certain atoms. Functional MRI allows visualizing brain activity by taking several images during a specific task. Nuclear medicine uses radioactive tracers, usable for example to detect in imaging tumor cells by accumulation of radioactive glucose.

nickname of Larry Smarr, a specialist in computational sciences and founder of the Calit2 Institute (*California Institute for Telecommunications and Information Technologies*) in San Diego. Although self-taught in the field, he is now endowed with solid knowledge in biology and is perfectly capable of interpreting the masses of data accumulated during his exams over the years. Larry has sequenced his genome, regularly analyzes the evolution of his intestinal microbiota, and performs numerous weekly blood tests, as well as regular examinations of his digestive tract by magnetic resonance imaging or colonoscopy.[5] The reason for this is that Larry has self-diagnosed as having Crohn's disease, a chronic inflammation of the intestine. Over time, he has acquired a deep knowledge of the scientific and medical literature on this pathology, of which he has become a true specialist. He is indeed the best specialist there is for his own Crohn's disease! Larry invites visitors to his institute to contemplate the detailed history of his biological analyses, projected on the walls of a room called *the cave*, but also to immerse themselves in virtual reality inside his intestine, thanks to a three-dimensional representation of his digestive tract, regularly updated in light of his latest exams! Larry the Transparent—who does not usurp his nickname in any way—even invited his surgeon to discuss his personal data to suggest how she should operate! Based on his experience, he encourages everyone to become the Chief Executive Officer of their health.

Larry's story, although unique, is not anecdotal. Today, many patients develop a detailed knowledge about their pathology, which they view differently from the doctor. Because if precision medicine aims to propose treatments adapted to the characteristics of each patient, the latter is obviously the best placed to explain to health professionals how his/her disease affects their daily life. In light of this expertise, patients of the future will not hesitate to express their expectations and beliefs to their caregivers. This idea of an expert patient is not entirely new. In developed countries, some patients who have overcome their addiction to alcohol and drugs or are living with chronic diseases such as cancer, HIV infection, diabetes, or multiple sclerosis can apply to certain universities for the "expert patient" diploma in order to advise other people suffering from the same condition.

At the same time, the progressive digitalization of medicine can only strengthen the role of patients in their own care. Thanks to applications for *smartphones* and connected wearable devices, they can now directly collect and transfer to their doctors data on their lifestyle and symptoms. Without a doubt, the patients of the future will feel more responsible for their health, their eating habits, and their potential risk behaviors. If patients like Larry the Transparent are still an exception today, they will be more the norm in the next 10 years. This anticipated evolution could materialize in the form of patients' management of their health, accompanied by the doctor and other health professionals, or even by *digital coaches* in the form of *chatbots*, providing personalized advice throughout their lives. Programs combining

[5] Colonoscopy is an examination performed under general anesthesia that allows the screening and monitoring of diseases located at the level of the colon, such as cancers, polyps, inflammatory diseases.

controlled nutrition and physical exercise could complement this adapted medical follow-up in order to stay in good health until an advanced age.

Beyond that, some patients perfectly informed about their disease can also express the needs not met by existing treatments on behalf of the community of patients suffering from the same disease. Such expert patients are now being asked to advise health industry professionals and regulatory authorities. Their opinions help, for example, to define the effectiveness criteria to be used to evaluate new drugs during clinical trials. These studies increasingly often include a measure of quality of life, which obviously reflects a subjective perspective specific to the patient. In addition, patients suffering from the same disease group together in associations that actively communicate on social networks, offering support to new patients in their care journey while educating them about their pathology. These associations also play an influential lobbying role in accelerating the development of new drugs and their evaluation by health agencies, especially when therapeutic options are limited.

Digital Twins and Virtual Patients

The management of his/her health by each individual is based on an optimal use of health data collected throughout life. It is clear that as of today, this information is still poorly structured and poorly shared among health professionals. The use of paper medical records indeed makes it difficult to exchange any new health data with all the caregivers involved in the patient's follow-up. In 2022, France set up a digital file called "My Health Space" with the aim of facilitating the smooth sharing of data with all health professionals, thus avoiding the sometimes-excessive repetition of tests and examinations, as well as the significant associated costs.

Beyond better exploitation of data, AI now offers the opportunity to create computer representations of each patient's own disease. By regularly updating these models, they could constitute valuable tools in support of personalized health monitoring. For this purpose, two types of disease models are envisaged: the digital twin and the virtual patient. The concept of a digital twin comes from the aerospace and automotive industries. It refers to virtual representation technologies used to train humans to interact with complex real situations. For example, airplane pilots are trained on 3D flight simulators to learn how to land on tricky airport runways in different weather conditions, taking into account the technical characteristics of different planes. This multidimensional simulation of physical reality by digital twins is now finding applications in many areas. The global digital twin market, which was USD 10 billion in 2021, is anticipated to be over USD 60 billion by 2027, with strong demand in health and pharmacy [3, 4].

Companies specialized in 3D simulation software, such as the French Dassault Systèmes, are already exploring the applications of digital twins in this sector. In health, the digital twin is most often used to simulate the functioning of a specific organ with its components and their interactions. In collaboration with the FDA, Dassault Systèmes has created a model of a living human heart, digitized by integrating anatomical data and documenting blood flow and cardiac electromechanical activity. By varying these parameters, it is possible to simulate the functioning of a normal heart, but also of an organ affected by different diseases. Other digital twins are being developed to simulate the structure and functioning of the human brain, lungs, and liver. Digital twins of complicated childbirths have even been made from images of the mother's pelvic cavity to model the passage of the child's head through the uterine canal.

Specific forms of digital twins, called "virtual patients," are today created using health data obtained from real patients, from their medical records, scientific literature, or clinical study results. These virtual patients are based on a set of biological and clinical parameters whose interactions are put into mathematical equations to simulate the impact of a drug on symptoms. A variant of the virtual patient is the "synthetic patient," designed by a computer from data collected from several real patients suffering from the same disease. The synthetic patient, therefore, represents a standard patient inspired by real cases but does not disclose any data allowing the identification of the original patients. All these digital twins and virtual patients have a great interest in health, as they are intended to represent the specific disease of the patient. As we will see later, these virtual models are starting to be used to complement real patients in the evaluation of drugs and medical devices.

In the near future, these virtual doubles will likely include not only the patients' molecular data, their genome, and their genetic susceptibilities but also their health history (results of biological and radiological examinations, follow-up medical visits, data collected by sensors worn by the patient), as well as high-resolution 3D images of their organs or even their entire body. This vision of a possible digital avatar constituting a virtual double of the patient clearly appears futuristic today, as the integration of all these data into a single model remains complicated in light of the insufficient calculation capacity of current computers. However, at the CES in Las Vegas in January 2023, Dassault Systèmes expressed its interest in developing a digital twin of the complete human body within about 20 years. In parallel, an international scientific consortium bringing together industrialists and academic researchers initiated the EDITH project in mid-2023, with the aim of developing models of virtual humans. When modeling technologies allow these digital avatars combining biological data and medical imaging data to be created, they will be able to be regularly updated throughout the patients' lives, in order to guide decisions concerning their health, simulate surgical interventions taking into account their anatomical characteristics, and predict in a personalized way the benefits and possible toxicity of existing, experimental, or virtual drugs.

The AI-augmented patient, therefore, covers the idea of a patient whose singularity is now deciphered with very high precision by medicine in the light of new technologies. But also a patient expert in his own disease, who has become a central actor in his health. This knowledge and this commitment of patients nourished by AI will allow us to propose treatments that are perfectly adapted to them. The reason for this is that in the mirror of a perfectly understood patient, AI offers the perspective of a drug whose properties can now be predicted before it has even been manufactured.

References

1. Esteva A, et al. Dermatologist-level classification of skin cancer with deep neural networks. Nature. 2017;542:115.
2. Topol E. High performance medicine: the convergence of human and artificial intelligence. Nat Med. 2019;25:45.
3. Marché des jumeaux numériques: croissance, tendances, impact du, COVID-19 et prévisions (2023–2028). https://www.mordorintelligence.com
4. Soudoplatoff. Le jumeau numérique en santé. Fondapol.org, September 2023.

The Predicted Drug

7

Making the Right Decisions to Design a Drug

The development of a new drug is a journey full of pitfalls. Projects are frequently stopped following disappointing results in clinical studies regarding the effectiveness of the candidate drug or the side effects it can induce in patients. These failures are mostly due to poor decisions made during the design of the drug. However, thanks to AI, the design of a drug can now be seen as a series of decisions that can be illuminated with different descriptive and predictive computational models, each requiring specific data sets. In particular, the important decisions to be made wisely concern the selection of a relevant therapeutic target, the choice of an adequate drug candidate, and the determination of the patients to whom the drug will be intended.

To guide human experts in these decisions, three applications of AI will be discussed below: disease modeling, identification of therapeutic targets, and the design and optimization of candidate drugs. A fourth application of AI, focusing on the evaluation of the performance of the drug or medical devices using digital twins or virtual patients, will be discussed in the next chapter.

In the first step, AI is used to establish a model representing the disease of interest, particularly with the aim of accounting for the heterogeneity of patients. This modeling is carried out from molecular profiling data obtained from hundreds or thousands of patients compared to healthy controls using the multi-omics technologies mentioned above. By integrating these large amounts of data, AI allows patients to be categorized into homogeneous subgroups based on their biological characteristics. Added to this are clinical data concerning the nature and severity of their symptoms, the more or less rapid progression of their disease, and the response to existing treatments.

By establishing a stratification of patients that reflects the complexity and heterogeneity of the disease, the model thus obtained allows the design of drugs adapted to each subgroup of patients according to their specificities. In fact, this modeling has now become the first essential step in creating a new drug from a precision

P. Moingeon, *Intelligent Drugs: How AI is Transforming Healthcare*,
https://doi.org/10.1007/978-3-031-91668-7_7

medicine perspective. For each subgroup of patients, the representation provided by AI of the disease as a biological system disturbed compared to normal allows the identification of therapeutic targets based on a very strong scientific rationale. Specialized computational analyses indeed lead to hypotheses about the genes or proteins important in the causality of the disease, then considered as privileged therapeutic targets. By making this choice based on a detailed understanding of the molecular mechanisms underlying the disease and by integrating a representation of patient heterogeneity, AI significantly increases the chances of success of future drugs directed against the selected targets.

Clearly, the targets chosen may be different depending on the categories of patients identified within a given disease. In this regard, a recent observation illustrates the additional interest of AI in designing more effective drugs, particularly for chronic diseases. Due to their natural history, which often spans decades, these tend to be heterogeneous, as demonstrated by the AI-based modeling studies already carried out. Moreover, in these chronic diseases, several dozen biological processes are often altered in many patients. To improve the effectiveness of current treatments that only target one—or a limited number—of these deregulated processes, it therefore appears that future therapeutic strategies will most likely rely on combinations of drugs. By providing a global representation of the molecular mechanisms involved in the disease, AI will allow the design of appropriate combinations according to the different subgroups of patients identified, based on a complementarity of targets.

In total, understanding patient heterogeneity, as well as identifying relevant therapeutic targets, are the foundations of any precision medicine approach. These insights indeed allow the biological characteristics of patients to be linked to the identification of appropriate drugs. As for designing and choosing drug candidates perfectly adapted to patients, AI now offers significantly increased possibilities.

Choosing Among Billions of Drug Candidates

After selecting interesting therapeutic targets, AI also proves useful in identifying drug candidates that interact with them. To design the initial drug molecules, we have seen that precise structural information is necessary. In 2018, the company *DeepMind*, a Google subsidiary, developed the AlphaFold algorithm, which, after several improvements, proved capable of reliably predicting the three-dimensional structure of proteins from their amino acid sequence, information much simpler and faster to obtain than determining the structure using complex physical methods.[1]

[1] Proteins are made up of chains of amino acids that form loops, folds, sheets, to adopt a three-dimensional shape that determines their biological function. The amino acid sequence of a protein is easily determined by mass spectrometry, this information now allowing to predict with good reliability the structure of the majority of proteins. In its most recent version, the AlphaFold algorithm allows predicting the structure in space of more than 200 million proteins, i.e., the majority of known proteins, derived from all living species. In October 2024, the Nobel Prize in Chemistry

Until recently, the screening of drug molecules that could bind to the target was carried out on robotic platforms, testing banks of tens of thousands of chemical molecules. Now, from the 3D structure of the therapeutic target, virtual screening allows the computer to predict the ability of billions of molecules to bind to the target of interest.[2]

This step results in the selection of a few promising drug molecules, which are considered as initial leads for the development of a new drug. To optimize these initial molecular versions, artificial neural networks are then used, which have been trained to develop algorithms capable of correlating the structure of chemical molecules with their pharmacological properties.[3] Today, deep learning allows the prediction of various properties of drug molecules, such as their affinity for the target, their interaction site defined at the atomic scale, and their activating or inhibiting effect. These computational analyses also help predict their absorption, distribution, metabolism, excretion, and toxicity characteristics. A truly revolutionary potential of AI is that it allows the parallel prediction of all these properties! Today, optimized chemical molecules possessing the required properties can be selected by computer in a space estimated at 10^{29} conceivable molecules (i.e., 10 followed by 28 zeros), without chemists needing to synthesize any molecule at this stage! Based on these predictions, only the chemical synthesis of a small number of promising drug candidates identified through AI will be realized so that their properties can be confirmed—or refuted—by laboratory tests. In addition to the significant reduction of necessary preclinical tests, the use of predictive algorithms greatly improves their chances of success in later stages of development.

In light of these already concrete achievements, health industry professionals are now decisively turning to AI to design drugs based on small synthetic chemical molecules. And this is all the more so as the short-term prospects offered by these new technologies seem even more dizzying. According to some experts, the quantum supercomputers mentioned above could allow for an even wider exploration of molecular space—up to 10^{150} molecules! To exploit these future possibilities that surpass the imagination, "competitive" artificial neural networks (*Generative Adversarial Networks*) operating in tandem can already design completely new molecules and even provide chemists with information on the recommended synthesis pathways to produce these novel molecules! In addition, the training of neural networks is now extended to the prediction of the properties of drugs based on other therapeutic modalities, such as synthetic oligonucleotides or biological molecules,

---

was awarded to Deepmind researchers Demis Hassabis and John Jumper for their work that gave birth to AlphaFold.

[2]A particular application of this computational modeling is the repositioning of existing drug molecules. By using databases documenting the known interactions between chemical molecules and proteins, one can indeed search for existing drugs that can be reused, as predicted to be capable of interacting with the therapeutic target of interest. This computational repositioning of drugs for new indications has been used to quickly propose potential treatments for severe forms of COVID-19 (see Table 1.1).

[3]For this purpose, the structures of chemical molecules are transcribed into binary language, in order to be analyzed using an artificial neural network.

such as monoclonal antibodies, peptides, recombinant proteins, vaccine antigens, and even bacteria derived from human microbiota.

These advances have begun to revolutionize drug discovery. For example, a completely novel broad-spectrum antibiotic, called Halicin, was identified in 2020 by AI in a few months. While it can be estimated that several thousand drug candidates have already been designed by the pharmaceutical industry with the help of AI, only about a hundred of them have so far entered clinical evaluation in humans. For these, the already observed benefit is that the discovery stage has been reduced to 2 years, compared to the 5 to 7 years previously needed for this phase. In June 2023, one of these drugs entered a phase 2 clinical study to begin testing its effectiveness. This drug, developed by InSilico Medicine, called INSO18_055, is intended to treat patients with pulmonary fibrosis. The first results of the clinical trial, made public in September 2024, confirmed an improvement in lung function in this complex disease, with a benefit obtained in relation to the dose of the experimental drug used.

These initial results strongly suggest that AI will significantly increase the productivity of the pharmaceutical industry by strengthening the scientific basis for the design of drug candidates and by accelerating the discovery phase. Numerous DeepTech companies specializing in the application of AI to the search for new drugs now offer their services to the traditional drug industry. With a significant anticipated improvement in the chances of success of these better-designed drugs in later stages of development, some experts are already talking about a probable wave of innovative drugs in the coming years.[4]

Health Industry 4.0 and Intelligent Hospital

Beyond its major impact on the discovery of new drugs, AI will also revolutionize their production and dispensation. It is indeed now part of the digital transformation initiated by the pharmaceutical industry and hospitals.

AI is one of the essential drivers of the evolution toward Health Industry 4.0, so named because it represents a fourth technological revolution in manufacturing activity. Throughout its history, the industry has indeed experienced two successive revolutions in the eighteenth and nineteenth centuries, respectively, due to the introduction of mechanical production enabled by the invention of the steam engine and then to mass production powered by electric and petroleum energies. A third revolution initiated in the 1970s was related to the use of computing and electronics to automate production. This fourth ongoing revolution is therefore fueled not only by AI but also by the Internet of Things, robotics, virtual reality, and cloud computing. Collectively, these technologies now allow the Health Industry 4.0 to generate and exploit large amounts of data in order to better coordinate activity flows and optimize the use of resources.

[4] International players specialized in drug discovery using AI include companies like Exscientia, InSilico Medicine, InveniAI, Recursion Pharmaceuticals, Schrodinger, Aqemia, Iktos. See also Stokes et al. [1], Punn et al. [2] and Jayatunga et al. [3].

In the pharmaceutical field, the first organizational evolution of the industry concerns the large-scale application of AI to support the discovery and development of new drugs with the predictive models mentioned above. To do this, industry professionals are currently setting up computational platforms that allow for the integration and analysis of gigantic amounts of data concerning diseases of interest, the biological processes involved, the known interactions between drug molecules and therapeutic targets, and the recorded side effects of chemical molecules. Using these different datasets, computational models based on AI are used, as we have seen, to support strategic decision-making in the discovery of drug candidates. The pharmaceutical giant Sanofi recently announced the deployment of AI-based solutions at all stages of the drug life cycle, thus reflecting a desire to integrate predictive computer modeling with traditional industrial pharmaceutical research and development activities, such as robotic chemical synthesis, high-throughput screening of drug candidates, automated preclinical tests, and large-scale clinical studies in humans.

Furthermore, AI is now being deployed by the Health 4.0 industry to improve the quality and production of drugs. Digital twins of industrial processes are used to compare different premises, equipment, and production methods by computer in order to optimize these parameters and increase productivity. Thanks to AI, the multiple activities related to drug production, such as raw material storage, active ingredient production, finished drug production, quality control, and batch release, are much better coordinated. The automation of manufacturing processes is also more synchronized with distribution and marketing operations. Virtual reality is also used to test new manufacturing processes and new equipment on a computer and to train employees in delicate production operations. Quality control at all stages of production is facilitated by the real-time acquisition and analysis of data captured throughout the industrial processes. From these data, algorithms developed by machine learning can predict production problems before they impact the quality of the drug so that the causes can be eliminated by preventive maintenance and thus avoid stopping the production chain.

In parallel, other technological advances are contributing to the modernization of the pharmaceutical industry's tools. The first applications of 3D printing to drug production have emerged, even if they are still anecdotal today. In 2015, the FDA authorized the marketing of Spritam, an epilepsy drug produced by the American company Aprecia Pharmaceutical, by 3D printing. The Chinese laboratory Triastek is developing an additive manufacturing method to print tablets for patients with inflammatory bowel diseases. This approach allows the thickness of the coating layers to be varied according to the patients in order to optimize the delivery of the active ingredient in a personalized way at the level of the digestive tract.[5]

The use of AI and these new technologies is identified as one of the solutions to remedy the shortages recently observed in many developed countries for a number of drugs. It contributes to improving the efficiency of the industrial tool, with the

[5]Across all fields, 3D printing technology is commonly used as a new mode of production for objects and materials, with a global market estimated today at 30 billion euros, growing by 20% per year.

new concern highlighted during the COVID-19 pandemic to secure the production of drugs and to ensure sovereignty in this matter for drugs deemed critical.[6] In the longer term, AI could transform not only the organization and operation of health industries but also the ecosystem in which they operate. In synergy with technologies such as Web3, the Internet of Things, virtual reality, blockchain, non-fungible tokens, and AI, it could promote the emergence of a biomedical metaverse. If realized, this health metaverse could in particular constitute a multi-dimensional collaborative space between large pharmaceutical companies and digital giants, particularly interested in extending their activities in the health field.[7]

In the same way, AI is now being adopted by hospitals around the world to improve their operations. The digitized transfer of data, coupled with AI analysis, is being implemented in major hospitals to better coordinate patient care from admission, consultation and diagnosis, care delivery, and billing to follow-up after hospital discharge. In developed countries, an organization based on AI and digital technologies has become the norm in the design of the hospital of the future. In Great Britain, the National Health System initiated in 2019 a modernization of the country's hospital structures largely based on a digitization of activities. In France, the Gustave Roussy hospital recently announced its digitization strategy for 2030, with the ambition to offer ultra-personalized treatments against cancer. This prevailing concept of the 3.0 hospital, also called the "intelligent" hospital, aims to transform the organization of care to treat disease faster and earlier, integrating molecular diagnosis, patient care, and personalized treatment. It also favors the evolution toward more preventive approaches to the disease [4, 5]. This ambition to create an intelligent hospital can rely on a digital health deployment strategy that promotes the use of new digital tools and telemedicine, as well as better exploitation of health data by using AI.

The expected benefits of the digital transformation of hospitals are multiple. For the patient, first, with better care, reducing waiting time and hospital stay, as well as personalized treatments favoring outpatient care. For health professionals, these new technologies should allow them to lighten the administrative tasks to which

[6] The policies of reducing drug prices in certain developed countries in recent years have indeed encouraged industrials to relocate the production of active ingredients to countries such as China or India, in order to reduce costs. The shortages observed recently in Europe concern notably old but nonetheless strategic medicines, such as antibiotics or anti-inflammatories.

[7] While the interest of GAFAMs in the field of health is not new, their initial ambitions have clashed with their lack of knowledge of the pharmaceutical universe, which is highly regulated. The GAFAMs are now approaching the field of health through partnerships with pharmaceutical giants, such as Novartis, Sanofi, or Johnson & Johnson, while developing their own projects. The Google Life Sciences health branch is a platform for evaluating digital technologies applicable to health, with investments in companies such as biotech Calico, DNAnexus and 23andMe, specializing in genetic data analysis, or the *Foundation Medicine* focused on molecular profiling of cancers. DeepMind, which also belongs to Google, is developing new drugs with the help of AI. Google's health subsidiary, Verily, has also launched a prospective study on thousands of healthy subjects equipped with connected objects to detect early signs of diseases. In addition to the medical application of its voice assistant Alexa, Amazon is also positioning itself on the distribution of drugs ordered online.

they are today subjected so that they can devote more time to their primary mission, care. We mentioned earlier the prescription or dispensing assistance software, which is now made available to caregivers. The same is true for the analysis of medical images by intelligent machines, which are now gradually deployed in hospitals to ensure a reliable and fast diagnosis and are automatable on a large scale. Robotic platforms are also used for the preparation of delicate treatments, such as chemotherapy. Other robots are directly involved in the provision of care, for example, in the form of surgical robots that operate under human supervision, but also in the follow-up of patients in intensive care. In China, a robot named Xiaoyi (which means "the little doctor") has been trained by absorbing the knowledge contained in many medical treatises. Xiaoyi even received a medical degree and is now used in assisting with care in a hospital setting near Shanghai![8]

On a societal level, the prospect of a future digitalized and robotized hospital using its resources more efficiently, thanks to AI, is also identified as a preferred route to lower health costs. In the next 20 years, it is estimated that the widespread adoption of AI and digital technologies could increase hospital productivity by 40–50%. This evolution will result in 90% of jobs in the health sector requiring a good mastery of digital technologies.[9] An advanced model of a smart hospital is that of Singapore. To increase the efficiency of its hospital infrastructure and minimize costs, this country has indeed bet on both the digital management of health data, the use of AI to exploit these data, and the omnipresence of robots in the provision of care and medication. According to the Bloomberg agency, Singapore's health system is today the most competitive in the world, considering three major criteria related to the cost-performance ratio, namely the average life expectancy of the population, the percentage of gross domestic product (GDP) devoted to health, and the average annual cost of these expenses per inhabitant.[10]

[8] The Da Vinci robot, marketed since the 2000s, has already been used in more than two million patients, notably for prostate removals, but also for heart valve repairs or renal and gynecological surgery procedures. These robots now rely on high resolution 3D imaging of the organs, tumors or lesions of the patients to be operated on, opening the perspective of very high precision augmented surgery. The question remains about the infallibility of these robots and human responsibilities in case of operative or post-operative problem.

[9] See the report of the panel of experts coordinated by Professor Eric Topol on the digitalization of the English health system (supra reference 22 in Chap. 2). Also see the report from the McKinsey Global Institute: *Artificial intelligence: the next digital frontier.* https://McKinsey.com/mgi/, 2017.

[10] With an average life expectancy of over 82 years and healthcare spending corresponding to 4.5% of GDP, or $2426 US per inhabitant in 2019, Singapore is ahead of Hong Kong (83.5 years, 5.3% of GDP, $1944 US per inhabitant) and Italy (83 years, 8.97% of GDP, $3032 US per person). In comparison with Switzerland, another reference country in health, the citizens of Singapore benefit from an equal life expectancy, a newborn mortality rate half as low, while devoting three times less of the GDP to health. The United States (78.7 years, 17.2% of GDP, and $8895 US per person) has a particularly costly health system, ranking 44th in the ranking of the 51 countries evaluated by the Bloomberg agency. France, whose health system has long been considered one of the best in the world in terms of cost-efficiency, is in the middle of these two extremes. The figures given are those of the year 2019, which do not take into account the impact of COVID-19.

References

1. Stokes JM, et al. A deep learning approach to antibiotic discovery. Cell. 2020;180:688.
2. Punn FX, et al. AI-powered therapeutic target discovery. Trends Pharmacol Sci. 2023;44:561.
3. Jayatunga M, et al. AI in small-molecule drug discovery: a coming wave? Nat Rev Drug Discov. 2022;21:175.
4. NHS. The Topol review: preparing the healthcare workforce to deliver the digital future. London: NHS Health Education England; 2019.
5. Vers l'ultra-personnalisation en oncologie, Gustave Roussy 2030. https://www.gustaveroussy.fr/

An Accelerated Evaluation of Drugs

8

Established Regulations and Regulatory Sandboxes

To better understand the peculiarities of the drug universe, it is necessary to mention, even briefly, the current regulatory framework in force before going over the evolutions induced by AI. The drugs differ from most common consumer products because they must satisfy multiple requirements of health authorities before being put on the market. Because of their impact on human health, strict regulation guides their evaluation, based on a double essential principle: first, demonstrate that the new drug provides a therapeutic—or preventive—advantage compared to any existing treatments; then, document the side effects related to the drug to ensure a benefit-risk ratio favorable to the patient. The current rules cover the development, production, distribution, and post-marketing monitoring of drugs. These regulations are established at the country level, but there are harmonized standards between Europe, North America, and Japan that guarantee the quality and safety of new drugs (see Box 8.1).[1]

[1] https://www.ema.europa.eu. *The European system of drug regulation*. These regulations, known as ICH, were established by an international committee (*International Council for Harmonisation of Technical Requirements for Pharmaceuticals for Human use* bringing together experts from regulatory agencies and the health industry. The ICH rules used by Western countries and Japan also serve as a reference for many other countries including China, eager to strengthen their own regulation.

P. Moingeon, *Intelligent Drugs: How AI is Transforming Healthcare*,
https://doi.org/10.1007/978-3-031-91668-7_8

Box 8.1: The Regulated Odyssey of a Drug

The journey of the drug begins with a phase of research in the laboratory, usually 5–7 years, to identify a promising therapeutic molecule. This step is followed by a preclinical evaluation of the drug properties in animal models or human cells. Regulations also require toxicological studies on animals (mice, rats, rabbits, or non-human primates) to assess the safety of the drug candidate before initiating trials on humans. These tests aim to detect potential risks of mutagenicity, carcinogenicity, local toxicity, or effects on specific organs or functions, including reproductive function. Considering these results, a decision is made to continue—or not—the evaluation of the drug by administering it to humans.

If the laboratory results are positive, the drug candidate is then subjected to strictly regulated studies in humans, after approval from health authorities. These clinical trials, whose framework is inspired by the Nuremberg Code and the Helsinki Declaration, primarily aim to ensure the safety of the volunteer participants. They require informed consent from each patient, based on a perfect understanding of the nature and purpose of the experiment.[2] Clinical trials begin with a phase 1 study, testing the safety of the candidate drug on a few dozen patients, gradually increasing the doses. Then come phase 2 studies, aiming to determine the effective dose on a larger number (a few dozen to a few hundred) of patients, then phase 3 efficacy studies involving large cohorts of several hundred to several tens of thousands of patients. The regulations also require, with few exceptions, specific trials conducted in children once safety is established in adults.[3]

In accordance with regulations, only pharmaceutical-grade drug candidates, produced in a controlled manner and perfectly characterized to meet specifications, can be administered to humans.

[2] The Nuremberg Code stems from a criminal conviction dating from August 1947 of Nazi doctors for their unethical experiments on human beings. This code brings together ethical principles allowing the legality of experiments on humans to be assessed, particularly emphasizing the voluntary and informed consent of the subject. It is complemented by the Helsinki Declaration, which sets out ethical principles for medical research involving human beings. These principles, adopted by the World Medical Association in 1964, evolve regularly as knowledge and technologies advance.

[3] In Europe and the United States, all clinical studies intended to support marketing authorization are registered in a public database. Their results, positive or negative, are published to be accessible to the medical-scientific community. A new European regulation (EU 536/2014) has harmonized clinical trial protocols and the approval process among member states since 2022, with the particular aim of improving the quality and transparency of data.

The pharmaceutical industry compiles all the results obtained during development in a file called the Common Technical Document. This file, now electronic, is submitted for approval to health agencies such as the Food and Drug Administration (FDA) in the USA, the European Medicines Agency (EMA) at the European level, or the National Agency for Health and Medicine (ANSM) in France. These public agencies are the actors who grant the pharmaceutical industry the authorization to market each new drug.[4]

As we will see, regulatory monitoring does not stop at market launch. The agencies carry out pharmacovigilance with the help of the drug developer and the medical community, collecting data on both the effectiveness and any adverse effects of the drug during its real-life use in the general population.[5] In addition, before its marketing, the drug is subject to an economic evaluation to determine its price and its reimbursement by public health systems in view of its performance.

The regulations specify to the health industry the prerequisites to be met for the marketing of any new drug. However, they can be a barrier to innovation, as technologies and regulations evolve at very different rates. There are, therefore, many situations in which these regulations need to be adapted. We have previously mentioned the adjustment of rules in emergency situations to accompany the accelerated development of anti-COVID-19 vaccines in 2020. Other adjustments include the easing of regulations for drugs against rare diseases or those that improve the treatment of serious diseases without a therapeutic alternative. The FDA has set up in such situations accelerated evaluation and approval procedures (*fast-track approval*) for drugs intended for diseases with a high residual medical need.[6]

A new drug showing moderate efficacy may be considered by health agencies as beneficial to patients who have no other therapeutic option. The recent US approval of Tofersen® for the treatment of Charcot's disease and of Aduhelm® for Alzheimer's disease, despite the limited efficacy in both cases, serve as perfect examples. A conditional approval is then often granted, which requires the drug developer to carry

---

[4] This CTD file consists of several administrative or technical modules that describe the composition and characteristics of the drug, the history of its development, the analytical methods used to characterize it as well as its manufacturing process. The results of preclinical, toxicological and clinical studies are also presented in detail in the file. Health agencies frequently audit the drug documentation, particularly verifying the integrity of the data. They can also inspect the premises where the future drug will be produced, as well as the quality assurance procedures put in place by the pharmaceutical laboratory.

[5] The information collected by pooling at the European level the monitoring of side effects allows health authorities to establish and regularly update the risk-benefit profile of all marketed drugs.

[6] The evaluation of the benefits and risks associated with a new drug varies depending on the severity of the disease and the existence of available treatments. An innovative drug bringing a significant benefit for a serious disease without existing treatment will have its side effects more acceptable.

out additional studies to confirm the marketing authorization.[7] The adaptation of regulations is also an effective mechanism to encourage the health industry to develop drugs against rare or neglected diseases. The granting of orphan drug status encourages such developments, even though commercial prospects are limited due to the small number of patients to be treated. Other regulatory incentives are commonly used to stimulate the discovery of specific drugs, for example, new antibiotics, in the form of a guarantee of exclusivity on the market or an extension of patent protection.[8]

Furthermore, regulatory innovation is imposed de facto for health products resulting from completely innovative technologies, such as drugs obtained from synthetic biology or nanotechnologies, which present unprecedented properties and risks. As we will see, new tools and methods based on AI also require specific regulations, most of which remain to be developed. To date, however, the intelligent medical devices and decision support algorithms offered to health professionals are already subject to initial specific rules. Regulatory agencies are currently considering establishing quality standards for the data used and strengthening the reliability and transparency of algorithms.

The rapid evolution of AI applications and new health technologies will require flexible regulation so as not to hinder innovation. To do this, the relevant authorities may, in certain situations, substitute the traditional regulatory framework, which is not very flexible, with an innovative approach called a "sandbox." This concept of a regulatory sandbox allows innovation players to deviate from certain rules in exchange for transparency toward the regulator, thus allowing mutual learning. The innovator can thus develop applications of its technology while being protected from certain legal risks, and at the same time, the regulator is in a position to better appreciate the benefits and risks associated with innovation in order to consider the most appropriate regulatory measures.[9]

---

[7] Alzheimer's disease is a neurodegenerative disease affecting 60 million people worldwide, without effective treatment, which results in presenile dementia. In 2021, the FDA registered in this indication Aduhelm® (aducanumab), a monoclonal antibody directed against a protein called beta-amyloid, developed by Biogen. The therapeutic benefit observed in a subgroup of patients appeared modest in the eyes of experts. However, the FDA authorized the marketing of this drug, given the significant residual therapeutic need. This approval was accompanied by an obligation for Biogen to further test the effectiveness of Aduhelm® in additional clinical studies.

[8] In the case of rare diseases, that is, those affecting fewer than 5 people out of 10,000 in the European Union, an orphan drug status can be granted, consisting of a specific marketing authorization procedure to facilitate their development, accompanied by a 10-year commercial exclusivity after marketing the drug. Regulatory incentives are also put in place to encourage drug manufacturers to develop new antibiotics. With an increase in the resistance of many bacteria to different families of existing antibiotics, the WHO indeed considers that humanity has entered a "post-antibiotic era" extremely dangerous, and that it is urgent to invest massively at the international level in public and private research in this field. Amabile-Cuevas [1]. See also on this subject the *Global Action Plan on Antimicrobial Resistance* and the *United Nation resolution on antimicrobial resistance*, both published in 2015.

[9] Regulatory sandboxes were initially set up in the field of finance to allow innovative companies to test new financial products or new business models. This particular form of regulation is now applied to many areas of activity, including health.

In total, regulations guide the continuous evaluation of drugs, taking into account their benefits and risks, but also, as we will see later, their socio-economic value. Health regulatory agencies are called upon to play a crucial role as innovation players by creating, in a collaborative approach with industry, new regulatory frameworks, both flexible and evolving, to fully exploit the applications of AI in health.

Disease on a Chip and Mini-Laboratory Organs

While AI allows for the design of an intelligent drug candidate on a solid rationale and with predicted properties, the latter must nonetheless be tested in the laboratory in accordance with regulations. Before clinical studies on humans, initial tests are conducted in preclinical models. Animal models, despite their limitations, remain essential today for the first evaluation of the distribution, metabolism, efficacy, and safety of the drug candidate in a living organism. These data collected in animals are used to model, by computer, the anticipated behavior of the drug in humans, particularly to predict its lifespan and estimate the necessary dose for effectiveness. In addition to the dose, these tests also help to define the administration schedule (single or multiple doses, intervals between administrations) and the route of administration (oral, injectable, etc.) that will be used in the first studies in humans.[10]

Other animal models are used to study the risks of toxicity, reprotoxicity, or carcinogenesis. In these studies, laboratory animals received increasing doses of drug candidates over different durations. The effectiveness of the drug is also tested, when possible, on animals with an artificially induced disease to reproduce human diseases, for example, different types of cancer, diabetes, or specific organ inflammations. Some animals spontaneously develop diseases comparable to those in humans, such as asthma in horses or muscular dystrophy in certain dog breeds. In addition, biotechnologies allow the creation of genetically modified animals, presenting diseases comparable to those in humans, thanks to controlled alterations of their genome. We mentioned earlier that transgenic animals, if a gene is added, are *knock-out* when a gene is deleted and *knock-in* when the animal's natural gene is replaced by a mutated or human version.[11] There are also "humanized" animals, reconstituted by human cells or tissues. For example, chimeric mice are created after grafting pieces of a tumor and/or the transfer of human immune cells. However, these models remain complex to implement.

[10] These pharmacokinetic and pharmacodynamic models are now carried out in rodents, but also in dogs or monkeys, which are more predictive of the fate of the drug in humans.

[11] These models have been made possible thanks to molecular biology technologies and more recently DNA editing mentioned above. Used at the embryo stage, these manipulations allow the design of animals in which the modification only affects certain organs, or only manifests at a specific stage of development. On an industrial scale, the South Korean company *Sooam* is conducting research on the cloning of large mammals, such as pigs and cows, which are genetically modified to create models of diseases such as diabetes, Alzheimer's disease or muscular dystrophies.

Although imposed by regulations on drug manufacturers, these animal experiments regularly provoke protests in many countries. However, despite certain limitations, preclinical studies on animals remain indispensable today for providing information translatable to humans about the properties of drug candidates, for example, pharmacological activity or the risk of toxicity. The use of genetically modified mice or rats has led to significant advances in the understanding of disease mechanisms. As such, these animal models are widely used to evaluate new treatments for many human conditions. However, it can be anticipated that the use of animals in drug research is likely to decrease in the near future. In 2021, the European Parliament adopted a plan to gradually eliminate the use of animals by promoting preclinical models based on human materials but also on computer simulations to evaluate the effectiveness of drugs, an initiative also supported by regulatory agencies.

An alternative to animal testing is thus to use human cells, whether they come from cultured lines, from patient samples, or from healthy subjects. For example, drugs that target the immune system can be evaluated on white blood cells easily isolated from human subjects' blood. Experimental treatments against cancers can be tested on blood samples from patients containing rare circulating cancer cells, without the need for biopsies. Human cells are also used in the laboratory to study the risk of toxicity of a drug. Banks of tissues and cell lines thus allow the determination of the drug target's expression profile in the human body. This information is useful for predicting an unwanted drug interaction and, consequently the risk of toxicity in specific organs. Other tests, performed after exposing human cells to drugs in a test tube, allow the evaluation of cellular toxicity, the activation of deleterious genes, or the secretion of unwanted proteins or metabolites. The effects of a drug can also be mimicked by specifically deleting the gene of the therapeutic target with CRISPR-Cas9 technology or by partially inhibiting its expression with *gene silencing* approaches to assess the functional consequences on different cell types. These cellular in vitro models have the advantage of being based on human-derived materials, but they are quite reductionist, documenting the effect of the drug only on a limited number of cell types and not on a complex tissue or organ.

Recently, two new types of preclinical models based on human-derived materials have been created to study the complex biological processes involved in diseases without resorting to animals. The first involves cultivating organoids in the laboratory from a patient's or a healthy subject's stem cells. These organoids are three-dimensional assemblies of cells that recapitulate the structure of human organs, for example, by forming a mini-brain or a mini-digestive tube. The second model relies on the printing of human biological systems, called "organ-on-a-chip" or "disease-on-a-chip." These biological "chips" consist of cells or tissues printed on a solid plastic support, then nourished by microfluidic channels containing substitutes for human blood. Depending on the biological materials used, these models can simulate the normal or altered functioning of organs such as the heart, liver, muscles, and lungs. These mini-organs, or diseases on a chip, are commonly used in pharmaceutical research to understand the mechanisms of diseases and to test new drugs.[12]

These various preclinical models, whether based on animals or human tissues, provide a multitude of data on the efficacy and safety of drugs. Today, AI is being used by the pharmaceutical industry to choose and design the most appropriate preclinical models for evaluating drug candidates, depending on their nature and supposed mechanisms of action. Of course, AI allows the interpretation of the large amounts of data thus produced to formulate hypotheses about the behavior of drug candidates in future patient trials. Finally, another contribution of AI that is generating major interest today is the prediction of the efficacy of drug candidates in humans using virtual patient models.

Computer-Based Clinical Studies

If the drug candidate successfully passes the preclinical evaluation stages, it can then be tested on human subjects. However, these multiple clinical studies are often very long, typically spanning a total duration of 5–10 years. Their cost is also very high, ranging from a few million euros for phase 1 studies to several hundred million euros for phase 3 studies. Furthermore, over 93% of the drug candidates entering human evaluation are abandoned due to disappointing results during these studies. By significantly improving the scientific rationale underlying the design of the drug candidate, AI will undoubtedly increase the chances of success during clinical studies.

In addition, AI is increasingly being used today to design and implement optimized clinical studies. The modeling of diseases discussed above allows for the documentation of the heterogeneity of patients and, thereby, helps to select those who seem judicious to include in clinical trials. Natural language processing with various tools—including ChatGPT—allows for the efficient analysis of a large number of medical records and thus identifies patients who will be eligible for clinical trials. AI combined with digital technologies has been widely used since the COVID-19 pandemic to remotely monitor decentralized clinical trials, collecting and analyzing data provided by sensors worn by patients in their daily lives. AI helps to interpret all types of data, for example, concerning pain, cognitive function, motor skills, or sleep quality, to discern signs of severity or disease progression. It is also useful for analyzing the positive or negative results of clinical studies, as well as for identifying biomarkers defining subpopulations of patients deriving a particular benefit, or on the contrary, presenting a specific risk, in reaction to the experimental drug.

[12] These organs on chips allow a detailed analysis of the proteins or metabolites secreted into the microfluidic channels by cells exposed to drugs.

Beyond the contribution of AI in the design and monitoring of clinical trials, it is, however, the possibility of predicting by computer the performance of a health product that is generating the greatest interest today. In one application, AI allows the modeling of patients receiving a placebo. This placebo, frequently used as a control in clinical studies, resembles the experimental drug but does not contain the active ingredient. Despite this, patients on placebo often report a significant improvement in their symptoms. This "placebo effect" is partly explained by the fact that care in a reassuring medical environment makes the patient feel better, even if they receive an inactive product. This is why it is necessary to include a placebo group in clinical trials to measure the real effectiveness of a new drug, beyond the placebo effect. However, thanks to AI, a virtual placebo group can now be formed from the data of real patients' medical records, whose progress under the study conditions—notably the follow-up duration—is known. The use of such historical controls is increasingly implemented in clinical trials that test the effectiveness of new drugs in serious or very rare diseases. Besides the interest, in such situations, of not administering an inactive placebo to real patients, this simulation method reduces the costs of clinical trials by decreasing the number of real patients included.[13]

In parallel, we have previously seen that AI provides first virtual models that can represent a specific patient's disease. These models are starting to be used to predict the effectiveness of not only medical devices but also of drugs. The digital twin of a living human heart, developed by the FDA and Dassault Systèmes, has thus been used to evaluate the effectiveness of *pacemakers* and *stents*, medical devices used, respectively, to stimulate the heart muscle and keep open a partially obstructed blood vessel. These digital twins, offering representations of healthy or diseased human organs, are mainly constructed from medical imaging data, and while they allow predicting a mechanical activity mediated by medical devices, they are generally not suitable for evaluating the effectiveness of drugs, which, by essence, act on biological processes. However, there are a few exceptions. For example, a digital twin was created by Spanish researchers to model in 3D the vascularization of a tumor in a young child from medical images. With this model, the researchers were able to correctly anticipate the diffusion of chemotherapy inside the tumor and thus predict the response to the drug, as well as the size and shape of the residual tumor after treatment.

However, to predict the effectiveness of drugs, the most common practice today is to use another form of disease representation, namely, the virtual patient. This type of in silico model is constructed from multiple biological and clinical data obtained from real patients suffering from a disease of interest. To build up the model, other data are taken into account, which concern the characteristics of the drug candidate, for example, its affinity for the target, its biodistribution, and its

[13] Frequently, the predictions of the evolution of the virtual placebo group are corroborated by the inclusion in the clinical study of a reduced number of real patients receiving a placebo.

lifespan in the blood, in order to predict its effectiveness on the symptoms of the disease.[14]

By varying these different parameters of the model at will while drawing inspiration from real patient characteristics, it is possible to create thousands of virtual patients and predict which ones could benefit from the candidate drug. For this purpose, machine learning is used to analyze the response predictions obtained for each of the virtual patients and train algorithms to identify molecular and/or clinical signatures distinguishing patients predicted as responders versus non-responders. These analyses are extremely useful not only for generating hypotheses about predictive biomarkers of drug response but also for setting a criterion that will help select real patients with a high chance of responding to the treatment during confirmatory clinical studies.

The computer simulation of a clinical study has thus become realistic, with the advantage of speed of execution and considerable cost reduction compared to real human studies. Moreover, this modeling allows the prediction of a drug's performance for an individual patient, even helping to define parameters to differentiate patients who will respond to the treatment from those who will derive no benefit. To date, these simulations are exploratory approaches, which are beginning to be considered as complementary to clinical studies conducted on real patients. As the reliability of predictive models improves, regulatory agencies will increasingly trust these data from in silico simulations. Already, the gradual acceptance of predictive models by major regulatory agencies, such as the FDA and EMA, is noticeable. These agencies wish to promote the 3 Rs rule, that is, Refine, Reduce, and Replace the use of animals and humans with simulation approaches in the evaluation of experimental drugs.[15]

In the coming years, the evaluation of a drug's performance will be done in a mixed reality approach, combining computer simulations on virtual patients with confirmatory clinical trials on real patients. Clinical studies will still be necessary, but they will be better designed thanks to AI, particularly by predicting the patients most likely to benefit from the drug, leading to a much higher success rate during the clinical development phase, which is particularly long and costly.

In the longer term, it will become conceivable to put new drugs on the market based mainly—or even solely—on evidence from computer models. Obviously, this

---

[14] This simulation method, called QSP (*Quantitative System Pharmacology*) models the dynamic interactions between the different components of the system (biological parameters of patients, symptoms associated with the disease and characteristics of the candidate drug) in the form of differential mathematical equations. These QSP models are recognized by regulatory agencies and are increasingly used by drug manufacturers in applications for marketing authorization, in addition to efficacy data collected during clinical studies conducted in real patients.

[15] In 2018, the US Senate encouraged the FDA to consider computer simulations as beneficial to public health, particularly because they promote personalized therapeutic approaches. The American agency, in consultation with industry, is currently implementing good simulation practices to promote these new methods in the evaluation of intelligent medical devices.

futuristic vision will depend on regulatory agencies recognizing the reliability of the evidence of effectiveness provided by predictive models based on AI. In this regard, the analysis of data from the real-world use of the drug on a population scale will be crucial to confirm the consistency of the observed results with the predictions of computer models during development. An application in which AI is already proving itself in order to ameliorate drug safety.

Safer Drugs: Thanks to AI

The evaluation of the performance of a new drug includes its effectiveness, but also its safety. This property is paramount in the eyes of regulatory authorities to grant a market authorization by establishing the benefit-risk ratio associated with the drug. In the case of a very effective drug with rare or minimal side effects, the evaluation is simple. But most often, a contextual analysis is necessary, which takes into account the nature and severity of the disease treated by the drug, as well as the residual medical need. If there are already drugs to treat this disease, their benefit-risk profile will be used as a comparator. In practice, it is important that the potential risks associated with the drug are identified in terms of their nature, their likelihood of occurrence, and their impact, and that they are appreciated over the long term, at the same time as the possibilities of preventing or reducing them.

We have seen that AI is particularly useful for analyzing all the data from the many laboratory tests, which allow the toxicity of drug candidates on human cellular models, but also their absorption, their distribution, their metabolism, and their excretion in animals to be evaluated. The often-automated implementation of such tests generates data in large quantities, effectively integrated by AI, which greatly enhances the scope of these initial toxicological investigations. During clinical studies, the distribution and metabolism of the drug are further documented with empirical data obtained in humans, unwanted effects are listed, and their link with the administration of the drug is confirmed or not. AI allows all this data related to the side effects of the drug candidate to be interpreted in order to accurately establish the safety profile of the drug before its marketing.

In the near future, it will be possible to go further by evaluating the risk of potential toxicity on virtual patients. By extending the prediction of side effects to cohorts of tens of thousands of virtual patients, it will indeed be possible to identify rare but serious events related to the drug, which are difficult to detect in conventional clinical studies, given the limited number of patients. Similarly, these models on cohorts of virtual patients will be able to predict harmful effects over the long term—for example, cumulative toxicity after repeated administration—not manifested in the more limited duration of clinical studies. Virtual patients could also be used to predict the safety—and effectiveness—of drug candidates in various ethnic populations, young children or elderly people, immunocompromised patients, or those with different comorbidities. These data on virtual patients, combined with machine learning to train predictive algorithms, will identify the biological and/or clinical signatures characteristic of patients specifically at risk after exposure to a given drug, under conditions (dose, frequency of administration, association with other drugs) perfectly defined. Ultimately, such information will be valuable in guiding the prescription modalities of the drug, as well as monitoring after administration.

In the meantime, AI is currently applied to the pharmacovigilance monitoring of the drug after marketing. Pharmacovigilance encompasses activities aimed at detecting, evaluating, recording, and preventing the side effects of drugs after commercialization. This monitoring of the use of the drug in real-life conditions is necessary, in addition to clinical studies, which, for the largest, involve only a few tens of thousands of patients. In this population-scale monitoring, AI is used to exploit all the information on the performance of drugs in order to update their benefit-risk profiles as they are used by an increasing number of patients. Pharmacovigilance is organized at the European level by pooling notifications of side effects collected by both manufacturers and regulatory agencies, as well as health professionals and patients themselves. AI significantly extends the amplitude of this large-scale surveillance by searching for weak signals of toxicity within the gigantic quantities of clinical, biological, and medical imaging data contained in the medical records of millions of patients.

Beyond that, semantic analysis algorithms have recently been used to perform multi-language analyses on messages shared on social networks (Facebook, Instagram, Twitter, YouTube) or in patient forums in order to detect rare side effects reported during these exchanges. Specialized companies in the analysis of these pharmacovigilance data have been created, with today's first confirmations of the significant contribution of AI in this field. For example, the onset of a flu epidemic can now be detected extremely reliably several weeks before being officially notified by the international public health surveillance system from simple informal exchanges on social networks between patients about their symptoms! Similarly, rare side effects of certain drugs have been detected on social networks, while they were not listed in pharmacovigilance registers. Today, the results of these language analyses by AI to detect weak signals of pharmacovigilance in interactions between patients are now compiled with the data from the WHO's Vigibase.[16]

Thanks to AI, drugs will be safer. In the context of precision medicine, it will be possible to identify subpopulations of patients for whom the benefit-risk will be favorable or, on the contrary, particularly degraded, thus inviting the restriction of the use to certain well-identified patients. Beyond the more reliable and earlier detection of drug safety signals by a vigilance system at the population level, AI will allow the creation of descriptive and prescriptive models, providing clues to implement the most appropriate corrective or preventive measures.

[16] Vigibase is the World Health Organization's database, listing tens of millions of reported suspected adverse reactions associated with drugs, which have been reported in about a hundred countries since 1968.

Reference

1. Amabile-Cuevas C. Society must seize control of the antibiotics crisis. Nature. 2016;533:439.

Part III

The Future of Medicine in the Light of Intelligent Drugs

A Personalized and Preventive Medicine

9

Matching the Patient and the Drug

If the shift toward precision medicine was taken about 20 years ago, it is becoming apparent that AI will significantly accelerate this evolution toward more personalized treatments. It is now conceivable to identify for each patient the appropriate therapeutic target, the most effective drug, its dosage, and optimal administration schedule, as well as the potential risks of side effects. By exploiting the data that, on the one hand, documents the specifics of the patient and, on the other hand, predicts the properties of billions of potential drug molecules, AI promises to match the patient with the optimal drug candidate. The models mentioned earlier, which simulate the patients' disease, will help predict the most appropriate drug for each of them, and evaluate their effectiveness and toxicity on a virtual double of the patient, thus paving the way for what we will call here a computational precision medicine [1].

The predictions made in the context of this new medicine augmented by AI will have to be confirmed by an evaluation of a small number of drug candidates in the laboratory and then in clinical studies in real patients. This AI-powered medicine will make available a large number of innovative drugs against most chronic diseases in the coming years. As mentioned earlier, initial observations already report an acceleration by AI of the discovery of new drugs in traditional therapeutic indications [2, 3]. Beyond this, the contributions of AI will, as we will see, allow us to explore new frontiers, such as enhancing body performance, stimulating cognitive abilities, or slowing down aging.

In its implementation, computational precision medicine will be deployed in two ways: stratified medicine and truly personalized medicine. Stratified medicine, which will be the preferred approach in the coming years, will offer an optimized drug to well-defined subgroups of patients based on shared characteristics. Molecular and clinical profiling will allow these patients to be categorized into homogeneous subgroups and to design drugs adapted to the molecular

P. Moingeon, *Intelligent Drugs: How AI is Transforming Healthcare*,
https://doi.org/10.1007/978-3-031-91668-7_9

dysregulations responsible for the disease in each subgroup of patients. Stratified medicine will be the norm for a long time to come, as it ensures the production of the drug on an industrial scale, with a pharmaceutical quality that meets the regulatory requirements.

In practice, stratified medicine requires that each patient be classified into a subgroup at the time of diagnosis, for which an optimal treatment has been specifically designed. As previously mentioned, this approach is already widely used for the treatment of patients with cancer after a molecular diagnosis has characterized the type of tumor affecting the patient, the presence of specific mutations, and/or the expression of immune checkpoints. From this categorization of the patient, various codified treatment protocols are applied, based on surgery, chemotherapy, radiotherapy, and/or immunotherapy.[1]

To be able to classify and follow patients during their treatment, stratified medicine requires the identification of biomarkers, that is, quantifiable biological parameters in the blood or identifiable from medical images, which reflect the severity of the disease or the anticipated response to treatment in the patient.[2] Some biomarkers predict the risk of disease before it develops. Others, called "companion diagnostics," are used to predict the response to a specific drug, which is then prescribed based on the measurement of this specific biomarker. For example, drugs acting on immune checkpoint inhibitors used in oncology are reserved for the treatment of tumors confirmed to express these molecules that can inhibit the patient's immunity.

AI greatly facilitates the identification of biomarkers that allow patients to be categorized for stratified medicine by analyzing very diverse molecular profiling data. In parallel, the first digital biomarkers, based on medical image analysis algorithms, have recently been developed to predict responses to treatments or the risk of recurrence in patients with certain cancers. In the future, even more efficient biomarkers will be developed in the form of multidimensional signatures combining biological, clinical, and imaging data, both quantitative and qualitative. These signatures will be used to make optimal therapeutic decisions based on an ultra-precise classification of patients in terms of the characteristics of their disease, as well as the prediction of its evolution and response to available treatments.

---

[1] These therapeutic protocols are defined after a multitude of clinical studies evaluating different treatments according to patient categories. First-line treatments (which have the best documented benefit-risk ratio in a defined subgroup of patients) are then recommended, followed by second-line treatments in case of tumor escape or recurrence, or even third-line treatments, etc. As an example of categorization, the MammaPrint test, which analyzes 70 genes, is now used to type breast tumors in order to predict the effectiveness of treatment and assess the risk of relapse in patients. The use of this test has shown that for 14% of patients, chemotherapy can be avoided after resection of the cancerous nodule, without negative impact on their survival. This test thus allows to avoid the harmful effects of chemotherapy to patients who will not benefit from it.

[2] Biomarkers are defined by the NIH (*National Institutes of Health*) of Bethesda, USA, as "*objectively measured and evaluated characteristics as indicators of normal or pathological biological processes, or pharmacological response to a therapeutic intervention*". Among the potential biomarkers that allow categorizing patients, monitoring the evolution of their disease or their response to treatment, we can distinguish those that define the disease (in terms of diagnosis, severity, prognosis) or guide treatment (by predicting efficacy or risk of side effects).

Toward Custom-Made Drugs

While stratified medicine already takes into account the specificity of the patient, computational precision medicine will, in some cases, take the form of truly personalized treatments. When a patient has a very particular biological profile, it can be difficult to classify them into one of the types of profiles defined during the modeling of a disease. In such circumstances, a custom treatment can be considered. The same will be true for patients with ultra-rare genetic diseases or those requiring therapies based on their own cells, for example, stem cells or immune system cells.

Although this custom medicine is now made possible—and sometimes even essential—with the emergence of new therapeutic modalities, it remains currently complex to implement. Offering a drug adapted to a category of patients as part of stratified medicine is becoming an established practice, but designing, developing, and producing a drug specifically for an individual is still a major challenge. In particular, these ultra-personalized approaches have the disadvantage of being difficult to industrialize and are very expensive. Interestingly, however, the emergence of 3D printing applications for producing small batches of tablets could offer a solution for obtaining truly personalized drugs tailored to individual patients while ensuring quality control. Regulatory requirements to obtain marketing authorization currently limit the number of drugs developed for a single patient, but there are nevertheless concrete examples, for example, in the context of gene therapies applied to very rare diseases (see Box 9.1).

Box 9.1: Mila and the Milasen

The story of Mila Makovec is remarkable in several respects. At the age of eight, this young girl was diagnosed with Batten disease, an extremely rare and rapidly fatal neurodegenerative disease. Mila showed difficulty in walking, progressive loss of vision, and significant seizures. Faced with this critical situation, a team of researchers in Boston sequenced Mila's genome, identified the mutated gene responsible for her disease, and then created a specific drug to treat her. In less than a year, this candidate drug was not only developed but also tested in the laboratory to receive FDA approval for administration to Mila. This drug, named Milasen, is a synthetic oligonucleotide that inhibits the RNA coding for the abnormal protein causing the young patient's disease.

This personalized treatment has slowed the progression of the disease, including a significant reduction in Mila's seizures. The development of the Milasen was largely funded by the Mila's Miracle Foundation through donations. Mila's story, published in 2019 in the prestigious New England Journal of Medicine, heralds future custom-made drugs to treat patients suffering from infrequent genetic diseases [4].

In addition to gene therapy that targets the patient's own genetic characteristics, there are several other forms of treatment that require personalized drugs. We have seen that some patients with cancer are now treated using their own immune cells, modified in the laboratory to obtain CAR T cells capable of effectively killing tumor cells. Similarly, stem cells can be induced in the laboratory from patients' skin or blood cells, then used as is or modified to create a drug. Moreover, some allergen immunotherapies are currently precisely adapted to the patient's particular sensitization profile to different allergens.

We can anticipate that, in the future, precision medicine will increasingly offer personalized treatments. A *Personalized Medicine Coalition* has been created, bringing together scientists, clinicians, industrialists, patients, and payers, all eager to promote these individualized treatments (www.PersonalizedMedicineCoalition.org). Advances in molecular diagnostic technologies and high-resolution imaging, combined with AI, will facilitate the detailed characterization of the disease specific to each patient. Sophisticated methods of multi-omic molecular profiling, currently reserved for medical research, will eventually be applicable to more patients and perhaps even to healthy individuals. With a comprehensive understanding of biological systems and detailed visualization of different organs, combined with information on lifestyle and environment, each individual will be able to benefit from the most suitable treatments.

Precision medicine accelerated by AI and computational modeling is underway to better care for each person, whether sick or healthy. This medicine is known as a "4P" medicine, as it is more personalized, participative, predictive, and preventive.[3] It is participative, as it encourages everyone to play a proactive role in managing their health, following the example of Larry the Transparent. The term participative also reflects the increasing contribution of patients in the design of new drugs tailored to their needs, as providers of health data and experts in their disease. Moreover, an expected benefit is that patients will be more inclined to follow a personalized treatment, which they know to be effective and devoid of side effects for them. But a particularly important dimension of this new medicine will undoubtedly consist in the emergence of predictive models of health risks that will allow the monitoring of each person, from birth to death. As a result, there will be a growing incentive to design drugs to prevent diseases before they manifest..

From Prediction to Preventive Drugs

Tangible signs of this predictive and preventive medicine, based on a better knowledge of patients, are already perceptible. By identifying in the genome sequence-specific mutations or polymorphisms known to be linked to certain diseases, predispositions to an increasing number of diseases can now be detected. A polygenic risk score based on more than 300 SNPs thus allows estimating the chances of

[3] Sometimes reference is made to a 6 P medicine, if we also add the improvement of the "Proof of evidence" and "Population-based" dimensions.

developing breast cancer based on a woman's age. In addition to cancers, other similar scores are being evaluated for various conditions, such as heart diseases, neurodegenerative diseases, mental illnesses, diabetes, and obesity. The *American College of Medical Genetics and Genomics* has compiled a list of 57 mutations associated with disease risks that can now be communicated to patients or their parents, as this information allows appropriate patient care. With the decrease in DNA sequencing costs and the availability of tests focused on the exome—the part of the genome made up of gene sequences coding for proteins—and not the entire genome, this list is set to significantly increase in the near future.[4]

Beyond these genetic tests, significant progress is being made thanks to AI in predicting diseases from medical image analyses. It is thus becoming possible to predict the aggressiveness of certain cancers without resorting to a biopsy of the tumor. In 2022, the Franco–American company Owkin introduced two diagnostic solutions based on AI image analysis, allowing for the prediction of the risk of relapse of early breast cancer after treatment but also to identify colorectal cancers with a high probability of responding to immunotherapy. These quick analyses allow refining the prognosis by classifying as risky a tumor previously considered of good prognosis, or vice versa. In parallel, American researchers have recently developed an AI application capable of predicting, by analyzing patients' medical records, pancreatic cancer 3 years before it manifests as symptoms! If these results are confirmed, this will allow a significant advance in the management of this type of cancer, which currently has a very poor prognosis in most cases, as it is detected very late.

As health risk prediction becomes more refined, medicine will become increasingly preventive, focusing more on the healthy subject. In this regard, predictive models based on AI offer the prospect of monitoring the health of each individual throughout their life. In a future in the making, human prediction could start as early as conception, taking into account the genetic heritage of the parents or even choosing the gametes used for fertilization. In the United States, companies already offer couples opting for assisted reproduction the possibility of selecting embryos based on polygenic scores. Although these choices are currently justified by the desire to prevent genetic diseases, it is likely that in the long run they might also be motivated by the selection of desired traits, concerning, for example, physical appearance or cognitive abilities, which obviously raises issues.[5] We can also anticipate an increasingly frequent use of genome sequencing and profiling of molecular newborns, combined with targeted diagnostic tests according to the family medical history.

Later in life, the individual's relationship with the environment will be documented considering their epigenetic profile, the composition of their microbiota,

[4]Among the 3 billion pairs of nucleotide bases that make up the human genome, only 1% corresponds to genes coding for proteins. The remaining 99%, once referred to as *junk DNA*, includes DNA involved in the regulation of gene expression.

[5]Turley et al. [5]. The prospect of predictive analyses leading to the selection of gametes and embryos could, at the societal level, result in changes in demographics, an exacerbation of inequalities, and a devaluation of certain traits.

their nutritional habits, their physical activity, and their exposure to pollutants, toxic products, and allergens. On a behavioral level, AI can provide information on the individual's psychological profile, for example, through the semantic interpretation of their written or spoken language or during exchanges with *chatbots* capable of determining their mood and even some of their intentions. Studies in functional brain imaging by magnetic resonance associated with AI are today being conducted to detect what attracts a person's attention—images, words, speeches—from an analysis of their brain, with preliminary results in thought reading that make existing lie detection tests look outdated [6]!

To globally evaluate the health status, initial algorithms have been developed, which predict with encouraging reliability the lifespan of healthy individuals. This field of research particularly highlights the predictive nature of the immune status, a rather expected observation given the central role of our immune system in the defense against infectious pathogens and cancer cells. In parallel, other works aim to determine biological age, that is, the objective measure of actual cellular and bodily aging, regardless of civil age. The length of the telomeres that protect the ends of chromosomes, as well as epigenetic modifications (particularly in the form of DNA methylation) or gene mutations associated with aging, are currently being studied to measure the state of biological wear.[6] The detection of proteins with an extremely long lifespan, especially in the brain, or the quantification in the blood of molecules reflecting metabolism and cardiac function, are other potential markers currently being studied to evaluate this biological age.[7]

With age, we have seen that the analysis using AI of genetic data, medical images, or medical records can predict the onset of an increasing number of diseases before they manifest. Other AI-based solutions will allow the early diagnosis of an increasing number of diseases or even establish a prognosis as to their future evolution or their response to treatments. We mentioned that voice assistants like Alexa can already diagnose certain pathologies, for example, COVID-19, by analyzing the acoustics of the voice and breathing. An application called Face2Gene, developed by the American company AICure, diagnoses certain diseases by analyzing the patient's facial features. This facial recognition-based device, trained on over 17,000 images of faces, can today identify hundreds of different genetic diseases, with a reliability of 91% [7]! In response to a declared health problem, algorithms will identify the optimal drug for the patient and predict their chances of responding to this treatment or the need to be hospitalized. If this is the case, other

[6] Telomeres are repeated nucleotide sequences that cap the end of the double strand of DNA making up the chromosomes. The company *Human Longevity Inc.*, created by Craig Venter, proposes to measure the decrease in the size of telomeres during successive cell divisions, in relation to the subject's age. The companies *Telomere Diagnostics* in the USA or *Length Life* in Spain market tests evaluating the length of telomeres in cells collected from saliva. Long telomeres could be associated with a lower risk of developing diseases or dying prematurely. However, there is inter-individual variability in the length of these telomeres, depending on the genetic background and exposure to environmental factors, which currently complicates the interpretation of these tests.

[7] Different expression profiles of these long-lived proteins have been observed in old animals compared to young specimens.

algorithms will help to determine their risks of developing various complications—for example, a nosocomial infectious disease—or of being admitted to intensive care, or even the probability that they will die in the short term [8].

According to the adage, every healthy person was, until now, an unaware patient. With individualized health monitoring throughout life thanks to AI, this will not be the case by 2050. If the scenario of the predicted human is still prospective—and can legitimately scare!—the first versions of the algorithms mentioned above already have a satisfactory predictive value on a population scale, for example, life expectancy based on the age group to which one belongs. However, with a limit, these statistical predictions established on a population remain random on the scale of the individual. Moreover, these predictive algorithms have been developed based on historical data, that is, from retrospective cohorts of individuals. There is no doubt that they will be improved with the continuous input of new data and advances in machine learning and computational analytics. Nonetheless, for them to be accepted by health authorities, their reliability will have to be established prospectively on very large cohorts of subjects followed for decades. Moreover, the parameters on which the predictions of the algorithms are based will gradually need to be made transparent—a requirement that more generally will concern any form of modeling by AI.

All these algorithms aiming to predict human behavior will only be truly useful if they can be associated with concrete interventional approaches to reduce health risks in the subjects concerned. When this is the case, it is conceivable that the analysis of all these health, behavioral, and environmental data will eventually allow us to establish a risk profile of the individual and then propose to them a *coaching*, for example, using voice assistants, fully customized in terms of medical monitoring, physical exercise, and lifestyle hygiene. Nutritional approaches may be suggested in the form of diets low in fats, sugars, and salt, adapted from an early age in order to reduce the incidence of future obesity-related diseases, such as cardiovascular diseases, diabetes, high blood pressure, and osteoarthritis. Other diets will be supplemented with vitamins, antioxidants, and probiotics, according to the specific needs of individuals.

In the long term, the ability to predict human behavior will encourage the development of drugs that prevent disease or treat it at a very early stage. The doctor will then be able to prescribe these preventive drugs based on a map of health risks identified for a given individual. However, it should be noted that the validation of the benefit of these approaches based on predictive tests-preventive treatment coupling will be complex and costly, requiring the observation of large cohorts of subjects receiving preventive drugs for decades. AI will therefore be useful here, on the one hand, to identify predictive biomarkers of risks in order to select the subjects to be included in these observational clinical studies, and on the other hand, to simulate in parallel by computer the long-term fate of virtual healthy subjects exposed to these preventive drugs. As we will see later, this AI simulation of virtual humans over a long period will also be particularly interesting for considering the development of future anti-aging drugs.

This evolution toward prevention guided by predictive models will have significant societal consequences, encouraging potentially directive and unpopular policies in order to modify behaviors considered at risk.[8] The emergence of preventive drugs will inevitably provoke resistance within a part of the population, similar to what was observed for COVID-19 vaccines. Despite these obstacles, the possibility of effectively intervening upstream, before the onset of diseases, will be favored in developed countries in the coming decades to address another major issue: drastically reducing health costs in order to ensure the sustainability of care systems.

References

1. Moingeon P, et al. Artificial intelligence-enhanced drug design and development: towards a computational precision medicine. Drug Discov Today. 2022;27:215.
2. Jayatunga M, et al. AI in small-molecule drug discovery: a coming wave? Nat Rev Drug Discov. 2022;21:175.
3. Punn FX, et al. AI-powered therapeutic target discovery. Trends Pharmacol Sci. 2023;44:561.
4. Kim J, et al. Patient-customized oligonucleotide therapy for a rare genetic disease. New Engl J Med. 2019;17:1644.
5. Turley P, et al. Problems with using polygenic scores to select embryos. New Engl J Med. 2021;385:78.
6. Tang J, et al. Semantic reconstruction of continuous language from non-invasive brain recordings. Nat Neurosci. 2023;26:858.
7. Gurovich Y, et al. Identifying facial phenotypes of genetic disorders using deep learning. Nat Med. 2019;25:60.
8. Topol E. High performance medicine: the convergence of human and artificial medicine. Nat Med. 2019;25:44.

[8] An adaptation of the diet of children genetically predisposed to obesity could be accompanied by regulation policies of the fast-food and soda industry, as is currently the case for tobacco or alcohol. It can also be anticipated that the prediction of health problems not yet manifested will influence the costs of health insurance and the obtaining of bank loans, particularly in the Anglo-Saxon context.

Stronger, Better-Looking, and Smarter 10

Improving Body Performance

The concept of using technology to enhance human capabilities has been popularized by transhumanism, a movement that emerged in the United States in the early 1980s. Transhumanism unites a diverse group of entrepreneurs, philosophers, engineers, and sociologists who advocate for progressive liberalism. Its proponents criticize the slow pace of natural evolution in adapting living beings to environmental constraints while emphasizing the potential of new technologies to radically transform humans, not only according to their needs but also their desires. Transhumanism, therefore, openly supports the use of a convergence of technologies to increase human capabilities beyond natural determinism. This idea encompasses the repair of bodies, stimulation of cognitive abilities, creation of new interfaces with intelligent devices, immersion in virtual reality, and extension of healthy life expectancy.

The transhumanist revolution thus appears both technological and conceptual, breaking the traditional relationship between man and nature, which is no longer figured as a model of perfection.[1] The declared ambition of this techno-philosophical movement to surpass nature may seem laughable; however, it will undoubtedly be a popular creed in this century. In reality, this Promethean aspiration has long existed, with thinkers such as Francis Bacon, René Descartes, and the positivists who have praised the merits of science and technology to free humanity from natural contingencies. The materialistic idea of the body as a machine, particularly exposed in Descartes' thought and reinforced by contemporary scientific advances, fits well with the transhumanist idea of continuously repairing its degradations with the help of technologies.

[1] The use of cosmetic products, cosmetic surgery, or contraception, which reflect the human desire to modify natural conditions, are compatible with this transhumanist stance. Indeed, nature is far from perfect, if we consider diseases, deleterious genetic mutations, or body alterations related to aging, which can be perceived as injustices from the perspective of the affected individuals.

P. Moingeon, *Intelligent Drugs: How AI is Transforming Healthcare*,
https://doi.org/10.1007/978-3-031-91668-7_10

However, it should be noted that the transgression of the laws of nature as envisaged by transhumanism is at an unprecedented level. It claims to modify the natural physical and mental abilities of human beings according to their desires, regardless of any health problem. Beyond the reservations that such an idea may raise, it resonates with the individualism and desire for unlimited choices characteristic of our postmodern world. It also echoes the need for transcendence inherent in the human species, particularly concerned for a long time with improving the performance of the body (see Box 10.1).

Box 10.1: Gaining a Second in a Century

The rigorous monitoring of performances in the main athletics disciplines began in 1912. Over the past 100 years, the recorded performances have been regularly improved, with similar trends for men and women, regardless of the sport, the duration of the effort, or the muscles involved. The progression of performances followed a relatively linear trend in most sports until 1990. However, from that date, it slowed down in many disciplines, suggesting more of a progression toward an asymptotic limit. Some sports medicine experts have hypothesized that by 2050, the human species will have reached its physiological limits in terms of power and speed in most sports. Some models even predict that by 2027, half of the world records will have reached 99.95% of their maximum limit [1]!

An illustrative example of this race for performance is the men's world record for the 100-m sprint, which was 10 s and 60 hundredths in 1913. It has been regularly improved by successive fractions of seconds during the twentieth century, to be set at 9 s 58 hundredths by Usain Bolt in 2010. This performance, achieved with a slightly favorable wind, is considered to this day as the upper limit of human capacity in this discipline.

The prophesying of a near attainment of human limits in major sports is, in reality, highly debatable, as it does not take into account the new—and future—possibilities of the medical and technological transformations of the human body. In fact, human body performance can be improved in various ways, including pharmacologically. In the world of sport, various medicinal substances—more or less licit—have long been used to increase performance. Historically, chemical doping with anabolic steroids was widely used in the second half of the twentieth century by Eastern European athletes to increase their muscle mass. Unfortunately, these "enhanced" athletes often proved to be fragile, with a reduced life expectancy. On the other hand, a study showed that cyclists who participated in the *Tour de France* over the past 70 years had an average life expectancy 6.3 years higher than that of the general population. This is explained by the genetic predispositions of athletes to effort, as well as their healthier lifestyle, even in the event of possible doping. Creatine, a permitted substance, allows athletes to temporarily increase their muscle strength. Growth hormones have also been widely used to optimize muscle power relative to weight, a treatment notably applied to Lionel Messi to enable him to become the world's best football player.[2]

Many athletes have resorted to erythropoietin or autotransfusion with the aim of improving the oxygenation of their muscles and tissues by increasing the number of circulating red blood cells. Salbutamol, an asthma medication, has also been frequently used to promote blood oxygenation. Amphetamines and beta-blockers like propranolol have also been misused by athletes to improve their concentration and manage their stress in competition. Narcotic substances, such as heroin, morphine, or methadone, have been used to alleviate pain during physical effort. Combined with amphetamines in what has been dubbed the "Belgian pot," these narcotics have been used by some professional cyclists.

More recently, the concept of so-called "genetic" doping has emerged, based on the possible use of gene, cellular, or molecular therapies to stimulate muscle cells or restore cartilage. DNA manipulation technologies could tempt some athletes to alter their genetic heritage to produce more erythropoietin or growth hormone. The technology of RNAs protected by nanoliposomes could also be diverted for these purposes, instead of a direct administration of the corresponding proteins, with the advantages of less easy detection and a prolonged duration of action. To date, no case of genetic doping has been reported worldwide, but the organizing committee of the Paris 2024 Olympics has taken the threat very seriously by setting up dedicated screening tests. The improvement of sports performances with substances that modify the intestinal microbiota (our second genome) is also envisaged. In this regard, the bacteria *Veillonella atypica*, present in large numbers in marathon runners, are of particular interest because they are capable of very efficiently metabolizing lactic acid, a by-product of sugar degradation during prolonged effort that causes muscle cramps. By avoiding cramps, drugs based on *Veillonella* bacteria could, in particular, increase sports performances in disciplines requiring sustained effort.

The question now posed to international sports federations is how far chemical, genetic, and technological interventions can be allowed in high-level sports without altering their essential characteristics. While chemical and genetic doping remain prohibited and the list of drugs allowed in high-level athletes is strictly controlled, the generally accepted rule to date is that new technological advances are acceptable as long as they are accessible to all competitors.[3]

---

[2] Upon his arrival at FC Barcelona, Lionel Messi was suffering from hypopituitarism, associated with a deficiency in the secretion of somatotropin, which gave him a frail appearance and small stature (1.40 m). Growth hormone treatment allowed him to reach his current height of 1.70 m.

[3] Another important lever on sports performance, sometimes called technological doping, involves improving performance through the use of new materials, devices, accessories by athletes. In recent history, the following have been successively banned by sports regulators: double-strung tennis rackets to increase the power of shots in the 70 s, grooved javelins to improve the lift of the device in the 90 s, polyurethane swimming suits to enhance glide in 2010. Among the technological innovations approved by sports federations are carbon fiber poles, parabolic skis, carbon tennis rackets, lenticular wheels in cycling, energy return athletic track coverings, and as of the Tokyo 2021 Olympics, certain high-tech shoes for sprinters.

In a completely different register, concerning sexuality, drugs like Viagra®, Cialis®, and Addyi® are commonly used to enhance sexual performance. Viagra® (sildenafil) and Cialis® (tadalafil) aim to treat erectile dysfunction by increasing blood flow to the penis. Addyi® (flibanserin), sometimes dubbed the "pink Viagra," was approved in 2015 in the United States to stimulate female sexual desire. Kisspeptin, nicknamed the "kiss hormone," could, in light of clinical study results obtained in 2023, stimulate libido in women and men suffering from hypoactive sexual desire disorder.[4] In parallel, a practice called "chemsex" is gaining popularity, which involves the consumption of psychotropic substances during sexual activities, often practiced in groups. Chemsex relies on the use of disinhibiting drugs based on new synthetic substances, such as cathinone, which increase sexual endurance.[5] This latter practice is not advisable from a health standpoint, as it can lead to dependencies, a depressive state, and social disconnection, as well as a risk of overdose that can lead to coma and death.

Still, concerning sexuality, in a more radical way, certain drugs are used to assist people wishing to change sex. In addition to surgery (vaginoplasty or phalloplasty), transgender individuals must take hormones for life to develop and maintain the secondary sexual characteristics of the desired sex. This hormone replacement therapy involves administering testosterone or female sex hormones (estrogens, GnRH agonists, progesterone) intramuscularly, orally, or cutaneously to allow transsexual individuals to masculinize or feminize their bodies, respectively.

Another application of drugs to body transformation concerns new obesity treatments. Obesity currently attracts particular attention from the pharmaceutical industry, with about 650 million people considered obese worldwide, of whom only 7% receive treatment. This condition is responsible for 5% of deaths worldwide and is associated with more than 200 types of complications, including type 2 diabetes and cardiovascular diseases. However, new drugs, some of which are administered orally, have recently shown remarkable effectiveness in treating obesity, offering an alternative to baryatric surgery. While treatments offered so far aimed to reduce the consequences of obesity, these new drugs are revolutionary because they promote weight loss and fat mass reduction. The most promising molecule in this regard is semaglutide, a GLP-1 receptor agonist, which was initially developed by Novo Nordisk under the name Ozempic® to treat type 2 diabetes. A more potent version, Wegovy®, was marketed in 2021 to help patients with diabetes lose weight. Eli Lilly's Mounjaro® (tirzepatide), approved in the United States as an antidiabetic, works in the same way by mimicking the action of GLP-1, a natural hormone that

---

[4] Pfizer's Viagra® and Eli Lilly's Cialis® are based on active ingredients that inhibit type 5 phosphodiesterase, thus acting as powerful vasodilators. The mechanism of action of Addyi®, marketed in the United States by Sprout Pharma, remains poorly understood; it seems to act at the level of central nervous system neurotransmitters to stimulate libido. The kisspeptin currently under development is also involved in the brain regulation of sexual behavior.

[5] The cathinones used are mainly 3-MMC and 4-MEC. They are often associated with poppers or molecules such as cocaine, MDMA (3,4-methylene dioxyamphetamine), methamphetamine, ketamine, GHB/GBL. Consumed orally, nasally or injected, these drugs induce euphoria and "empathy", greatly enhancing physical sensations.

regulates appetite by stimulating the feeling of satiety. These drugs allow obese people to lose between 15% and 21% of their weight, compared to a 25% reduction typically observed after invasive bariatric surgery. The estimated market for this class of drugs was USD 4 billion in 2022. With the potential to reduce all obesity-related diseases, it could exceed USD 50 billion by 2030![6]

And what about AI in all this? AI modeling of metabolic diseases, so named because they are particularly related to the dysregulation of biological processes associated with sugar or fat metabolism, will undoubtedly help identify new therapeutic targets to design new drugs. It could allow for personalized obesity treatments, depending on the patient's specifics and eating habits. AI can also be used by each individual hesitating between different body reshaping approaches to create, from an original photograph, remarkably realistic three-dimensional parametric models of their transformed body, operating at will, distortions in terms of weight, size, and musculature.[7] In line with the transhumanist credo of transforming one's body according to one's desires, these models built *à la carte* by AI will guide the choices of those who, in the future, will be tempted to submit their bodies to genetic manipulations, regenerative medicine based on stem cells, drugs from synthetic biology, 3D tissue printing, intelligent prosthetics, or even various forms of hybridization with machines.

There is no doubt that with all the opportunities offered by technologies, more and more individuals will be eager to transform their bodies during this century. Particularly in light of this other essential concern of the human species, improving physical appearance.

Esthetics and Precision Cosmetology

Over time, esthetic standards evolve, but the quest for beauty remains a constant in human history. Each of us is influenced to varying degrees by the beauty standards valued by society at a given time. Beyond socially constructed preferences, neurobehavioral sciences have shown that the human species has an innate perception of certain characteristics considered harmonious. Humans are, for example, sensitive to the symmetry of features and an "average" appearance, favoring neutral faces rather than overly marked features. Natural evolution has also favored the ability to quickly detect signs of youth, health, and fertility to identify optimal partners for reproduction. Sexual differentiation characteristics, body odor, the way of moving, the texture of the skin, and hair are particularly appreciated. This attraction to what

[6] Morgan Stanley. *Unlocking the obesity challenge: a $50 Bn market*. July 2022. GLP1 (Glucagon-like peptide) is a hormone that stimulates the production of insulin and inhibits the production of glucagon. Semaglutide also acts at the level of the hypothalamus by inducing satiety. Wegovy® is prescribed to treat patients with a body mass index of 35 kg per m^2 or higher, in combination with a low-calorie diet and physical activity.

[7] Approaches based on artificial neural networks with the evocative title, NeuralReshaper, allow for the generation of comparative "before and after" images of the envisaged body transformation.

we consider beautiful has led to the notion of an "esthetic brain," involving complex neurosensory circuits.[8]

While for a long time natural body characteristics were little modifiable, the use of beauty products and cosmetic surgery now allows everyone to transform their appearance beyond what is given by nature. Who could question this ordinary and legitimate desire to want to appear at their best by mitigating the effects of time? The annual global beauty product market, including makeup, dermocosmetics, hygiene and care products, hair products, and perfumes, exceeds USD 800 billion, with a steady growth of about 5% per year.[9] Beyond these traditional cosmetic products, esthetic medicine is turning toward biological products and new technologies. Botox, for example, based on a powerful toxin produced by the bacterium *Clostridium botulinum*, is now widely used to reduce wrinkles by relaxing facial muscles. Hyaluronic acid helps to fill in wrinkles to reduce them. Cryolipolysis, which involves cooling tissues to eliminate body fat, also known as *CoolSculpting*, is applied as a slimming technique for targeted parts of the body.

However, the most interesting direction in cosmetology is the one that echoes contemporary medicine, that is, a personalized approach to care, facilitated by AI. The latter now allows the collection and analysis of large amounts of data specific to each individual, concerning the texture of their skin, the nature of their hair, or the aging of their tissues, in order to offer them perfectly adapted body care. Cosmetic companies are interested in genetic testing to predict the future skin aging level of their clients, particularly by assessing their ability to metabolize collagen or their resistance to oxidative stress. This evolution toward precision cosmetology, thanks to AI, also encompasses understanding the psychosociological characteristics of the client, allowing for targeting their receptivity to various marketing messages. Computer modeling is already used to design new products and predict their success among different categories of customers. AI is, for example, used by the perfume industry to integrate the characteristics of thousands of ingredients and then to model on the computer the millions of possible formulas by combining these components to create new products [2].

In parallel, advances in living technologies offer sometimes surprising models to evaluate the effectiveness of new cosmetic products. For example, the Riken Institute in Japan recently created a small integumentary system from human stem cells, including the skin, hair, and sweat glands. This mini-organ—which could be generated for each individual—works perfectly and can even secrete sweat in a test tube! It could thus be used in the laboratory to test in a personalized way the effect

[8] When we look at a face, the signals collected by the eye are transmitted to the occipital lobe, located at the back of the brain, which immediately interprets the information concerning facial expression, gaze, position of the lips… Other areas of the brain analyze this information in terms of emotional status. Faces perceived as beautiful stimulate the dopaminergic areas of the brain, such as the nucleus accumbens, which is responsible for our sensations of pleasure. Another region, the amygdala, is instead activated by signals deemed frightening (*fear factors*), for example the sight of snakes or insects. These different brain areas contribute to establishing a judgment of trust or mistrust.

[9] Source: Zion Market Research.

of cosmetic or body hygiene products. In this same perspective of personalization, virtual reality is used to overlay different types of makeup, lipstick, nail polish, handbags, or clothes on a customer's photo to check their harmony with the color of her skin or hair. A field of research called "hormonal beauty" even aims to offer customers makeup products adapted to their menstrual cycle!

Clearly, the radical transformation of appearance using cosmetic surgery is, by nature, a personalized intervention. New technologies now allow for very precise responses to the needs and anatomical characteristics of the individual. From tomography images, it is possible to obtain a very detailed 3D representation of a person's face or organs, including their bones, nerves, and muscles. For repair purposes, we have seen that it is possible to print in three dimensions inert matrices from plastic, heat-resistant metal, or even ceramics that can withstand higher temperatures. 3D printing of biocompatible materials allows the production of bones to modify or reconstruct a jaw, a chin, a forehead, or, more generally, reshape a face. It is highly likely that the use of these approaches in esthetic medicine is set to grow significantly in the coming years.

From Cognitive Enhancement to Brain-Computer Hybridization

Since the middle of the twentieth century, various categories of drugs have been available to treat brain disorders. Among these psychotropic drugs, we can mention neuroleptics, anxiolytics, antidepressants, sleeping pills, mood regulators. Collectively, these drugs have improved the management of many mental illnesses, which affect more than one in eight people worldwide and whose frequency, according to current forecasts, is set to increase globally. In parallel, the unmet medical needs remain very significant for neurodegenerative diseases, which are also set to increase with the aging of the population. Alzheimer's, Parkinson's, Huntington's, or Charcot's diseases result from the destruction of neurons in different parts of the brain, altering cognitive and/or motor functions depending on the case. Truly effective treatments for these complex diseases remain to be developed; with, however, new advances have recently been made in these indications, notably thanks to oligonucleotides and monoclonal antibodies, with drugs approved in recent years in the United States, such as Tofersen for Charcot's disease and Leqembi and Kisuma for Alzheimer's disease.

This therapeutic field should, in the coming years, benefit greatly from the progress made in our understanding of the human brain and the possibility of extending or reproducing some of its functionalities with the help of intelligent machines. Currently, AI is being used to design and develop new drugs against neurodegenerative diseases. Models of most of these diseases are now established, which allows the identification of promising new therapeutic targets. Digital twins of the human brain, healthy or pathological, as well as virtual patients representative of Alzheimer's disease, have been created, which will help to predict by computer the effectiveness of future drugs. In combination with new therapies targeting mutated or dysregulated genes, notably with the help of synthetic oligonucleotides, major advances are expected in the next 10 years in the management of these neurological diseases.

Beyond this, there is growing interest in the ambition made popular by science fiction books, but also by transhumanists, to enhance the cognitive abilities of perfectly healthy individuals. The prospect of administering drugs that stimulate intelligence to non-sick individuals is controversial, given the risk of creating inequalities in intellectual abilities within the population. However, in order to improve cognitive performance, many drugs and psychotropic substances are already being diverted from their initial use. Students frequently use psychostimulants such as Adderall®, Provigil® (modafinil), or Ritalin® (methylphenidate) to increase their productivity, concentration, and memory by staying awake. Hallucinogenic psychotropics such as psilocin, psilocybin, LSD, GHB, and ketamine are often used illicitly to alter behaviors. Moreover, there is currently a pronounced interest in the *cognitive enhancement* of humans using new pharmacological molecules in development, called nootropics. The aim of these substances is to improve the intellect and motivation without causing side effects.[10]

While waiting for a proven benefit from these drug molecules, medical devices are currently being considered to increase human brain functions. Some of these devices, which allow electrostimulation of the prefrontal cortex, are very popular among video game users.[11] Other methods, such as transcranial magnetic or electrical stimulation, deep brain stimulation, and *neurofeedback*, are capable of modifying brain activity in real time. However, their effectiveness varies among individuals, and their long-term effects on health are poorly understood. They can, in particular, create risks of addiction or sleep disruption, with potentially harmful effects on mental health and memory.[12] Deep brain stimulation after the implantation of electrodes in the brain is now used to treat patients suffering from epilepsy, obsessive-compulsive disorders, severe depression, or Parkinson's disease.

The U.S. Department of Defense is interested in a brain implant designed to stimulate the hippocampus, an important region of the brain in memorization, with the aim of restoring memory in soldiers traumatized by wars in Afghanistan or Iraq. If successful, this approach could be applied to patients with Alzheimer's disease or other neurodegenerative disorders. In the longer term, other ongoing research concerns the development of brain implants to connect the human brain and the computer. Institutes such as Max Planck in Munich and Caltech in California, as well as the company Neuralink, founded by Elon Musk in 2016, are working on electronic

[10] Apart from these drug approaches, there are "gentle" brain programming and stimulation methods that involve the use of images, sounds, or positive representations, such as neuro-linguistic programming. Popular authors such as Tony Robbins have written numerous books on personal development using these methods, with evocative titles such as *Unlimited power* (Free Press, 1986) or *Awaken the giant within* (Free Press, 1991).

[11] Such devices are marketed in the USA by companies such as Foc.us and Thync. They are curiously not regulated by the FDA.

[12] See Opinion 122 of the French Consultative Ethics Committee. *Recours aux techniques biomédicales en vue de neuro-amélioration chez la personne non malade: enjeux éthiques*. 2013.

chips inserted into the brain to improve human brain functions and create brain-computer interfaces. If these approaches prove effective, they will open new frontiers in the possible interactions between human intelligence and AI, the scope of which is still difficult to imagine.[13]

These ongoing developments make this concept, often discussed in science fiction, of a hybridization between man and machine in the form of a *cyborg* (contraction of *cybernetic organism*) more realistic. Unlike a fully artificial robot programmed by humans, the *cyborg* resulting from the fusion of a human and a machine is presented in futuristic novels as an autonomous being.[14] More recently, the term *cyborg* has been used to describe a human being who integrates a mechanical or electronic part. This can therefore include sensu stricto individuals who receive prostheses or implants for medical purposes. In the future, *cyborgs* could present themselves as true hybrid creatures between man and machine. Kevin Warwick, a cybernetics specialist and professor at the University of Reading in England, argues that modifying the human body by adding or inserting artificial elements does not raise any particular ethical issues, even if it significantly alters physical performance and can blur the boundary between man and machine. According to this expert, there are ethical problems only if the machine or the prosthesis, directly connected to the human brain, can change the mental state, consciousness, or behavior of the human. All boundaries that humanity has already begun to explore [3].

References

1. Berthelot G et al. La fin du Citius: La progression des records du monde durant l'ère olympique annoce l'épilogue d'une brêve quête ultra-physiologique. www.insep.eu/fr/activites/recherche-medicales/irmes-presse/Documents; 2011.
2. Les Échos Week-End. L'intelligence artificielle a-t-elle du nez? 12 Feb 2021.
3. Warwik K. Cyborg morals, cyborg values, cyborg ethics. Ethics Inform Technol. 2003;5:131.

[13] See the Neuralink video (*Monkey MindPong* youtube.com) showing a monkey playing the video game of ping-pong by activating its racket with its thought. This modernized game has been aptly named Mind Pong!

[14] The term "cybernetics" was created in 1947 by Norbert Wiener to describe the study of information and communication mechanisms in complex natural or artificial systems, with a particular interest in the control of machines by man. This field is considered very important in the emergence of robotics and artificial intelligence as we know them today.

11 Death of Death and Rejuvenation Pills

Technological Assaults Against Death

Human life, as Woody Allen aptly summarizes, is a deadly disease that is sexually transmitted. Aging and death are embedded in our biology from birth; they are an integral part of life. Aging is defined as an increase in the risk of death over time; this risk doubles every 8 years for our species. Every day, about 150,000 people die in the world, of which 100,000 die due to aging, directly linked to a notable increase in cancers, neurodegenerative diseases, and heart diseases. On a philosophical level, death is legitimized as a natural process, inevitable and necessary to preserve the species by eliminating the old individuals. Despite the apparent wisdom of this precept, it could be questioned for a part of the population as we progress in this century. With the power of new technologies, some might indeed consider death on an individual level not as a fatality inherent to the human condition but more as an injustice to fight.

In his very particular relationship with death, it is interesting to mention here Ray Kurzweil, a professor at the Massachusetts Institute of Technology in Boston and an avowed transhumanist. This physicist, born on February 12, 1948, takes a daily mix of 200 tablets of vitamins, antioxidants, and anti-inflammatories to fight against aging![1] To grasp the thinking of this singular visionary, let's remember that if one lives today in a developed country, one can hope to gain 2 to 3 months of life expectancy every year. According to Kurzweil, joined in this by the Harvard biologist George Church and entrepreneur Peter Diamandis, within one or two decades, we could, thanks to advances in medicine, gain a whole year of life every year!

[1] In addition to the unproven effectiveness of such self-medication, mixtures of drugs not documented by dedicated studies are obviously to be avoided. Interactions between drugs can indeed reveal toxicities or reduce their effectiveness compared to the intake of individual drugs.

P. Moingeon, *Intelligent Drugs: How AI is Transforming Healthcare*,
https://doi.org/10.1007/978-3-031-91668-7_11

Strengthened by this conviction, Kurzweil and his supporters aim to cross these few necessary years to finally access this promise of longevity, with the ultimate ambition of reaching an age where technologies will allow us to download the human brain onto the hard drive of a computer...

Let's recall here that the transhumanists, not stingy with ambitious promises on the subject, have loudly proclaimed that a convergence of new technologies will allow us to reach "the death of death" by 2045 [1]! This ambition, supported with conviction by figures such as the Russian billionaire Dmitry Itskov and numerous personalities from Silicon Valley, has, of course, no chance of materializing and is, in fact, totally unrealistic. One reason for this is that, as we will explain later, we are barely at the beginning of understanding the biological mechanisms of aging to design the first drugs aimed at slowing down the wear and tear of the body. Before we delve into this more realistic project, we will review some astonishing approaches seriously considered by the transhumanist movement to defy death.

After death, an a priori legitimate strategy is to preserve the body of the deceased as best as possible, hoping to bring it back to life when a treatment for the cause that led to death has been discovered. More than 5000 years ago, embalming and mummification techniques based on natural resins were developed in ancient Egypt. Today, the focus is on cryopreservation in liquid nitrogen at −196 °C. The American company Alcor offers this method called cryonics, which involves quickly freezing all or part of the body to prevent its decomposition. In 2016, a young British patient with terminal cancer expressed her wish to be cryopreserved in anticipation of a treatment becoming available in the future. In early 2021, this Arizona-based company claimed more than 180 "patients," the term here referring to deceased people immersed in liquid nitrogen, with over 1300 "members" having made a reservation for this procedure "when the time comes." However, it should be noted that post-mortem regeneration is currently impossible and will remain so for a long time. Although we can freeze cells and even very simple organisms such as worms in the laboratory, we are still unable to do the same for multicellular organisms as complex as human bodies, to consider thawing them while preserving their vitality.[2]

Another approach to defeating death considered by some scientists would be to clone deceased individuals from one of their cells, thus accessing their complete genetic heritage.[3] The cloning of higher animals is technologically possible and was first successful in 1996 with the famous sheep Dolly, derived from a cell from the

[2] Perhaps future technologies will be able to maintain still living bodies in a state of hibernation for long periods? These hibernation and torpor mechanisms are very studied in the animal world. They consist of a resting of the organism while maintaining a low residual metabolic activity, which allows the animal to recover all its vital functions, when environmental conditions are favorable. These biological mechanisms are currently studied using molecular profiling techniques comparing animals in a state of hibernation with others in normal living conditions.

[3] Each cell in the body, for example from the blood or skin, contains the entire genetic heritage of the individual. However, the 23,000 genes express themselves differently depending upon the tissue, due to regulatory mechanisms that allow cells from different organs to perform distinct functions.

mammary gland of an adult sheep. However, Dolly proved to be fragile and died prematurely, probably because the biological clock of the cell used for cloning had not been reset in the process.[4] The feasibility of cloning from the cell of an adult individual to obtain a perfectly healthy human being is therefore totally uncertain. Moreover, the cloning of a human being is to this day strictly forbidden for obvious ethical reasons. Although intentions to clone humans have been expressed by the Raelian Church, as well as by researchers Richard Seed and Severino Antinori, they have been unanimously condemned by the scientific community and have never been implemented. However, in mid-2023, three independent research teams announced the production of human embryos from embryonic stem cells. These so-called "synthetic" embryos, created without fertilization, developed normal morphological characteristics up to 14 days, the maximum duration allowed for the culture of human embryos in the laboratory. If these studies aimed to obtain models for studying early human development, perhaps they will one day encourage the use of this type of approach to clone a human being?[5]

In an even more futuristic vision to fight against death, some researchers like Kurzweil and the transhumanist philosopher Nick Bostrom propose to save the content of an individual's brain by downloading it onto a computer or into the *cloud*. This method, called *upload*, raises great skepticism, as it transgresses the knowledge of contemporary neurobiology. Although we can save documents on digital

---

[4] To achieve cloning, the nucleus of a cell (containing the genetic heritage) taken from an adult ewe named Geniees was reinjected into the ovum of another ewe named Belinda, whose nucleus had been previously removed. This reconstituted ovum produced an embryo that gave birth to an animal genetically identical to Geniees, which the researchers called Dolly. Appearing healthy, Dolly lived just over 6 and a half years (between 1996 and 2003). She died prematurely, affected by arthritis problems and respiratory difficulties. The potential explanation for this limited lifespan is that Dolly was cloned from a cell of an adult animal, essentially constituting her biological age at birth. Her naturalized body is now on display at the National Museum of Scotland, in Edinburgh.

[5] Oldak et al. [2]. While cloning theoretically allows for the creation of an individual genetically identical to the donor of the original cell, the clone will indeed resemble the donor like a homozygous twin, but the expression of its genetic heritage and its psychology, both shaped in part by its experiences, will be different from those of the original "twin". In many countries, legislation distinguishes between reproductive cloning (aiming to reproduce identical individuals) and therapeutic cloning (to produce embryos as a source of stem cells for medical purposes). The Charter of Fundamental Rights of the European Union adopted in 2000 prohibits the reproductive cloning of human beings. The United Nations General Assembly reiterated in 2005 the prohibition of this cloning, including for therapeutic purposes. The duplication of pets by cloning is, however, now commonly performed by the company Sooam, founded by South Korean professor Hwang Woo-Suk. In 2004, this South Korean professor became a celebrity in the scientific world by announcing that he had cloned a human embryo to produce stem cells, before admitting, 2 years later, that his data were falsified… Sooam, specializing in the cloning of pets and livestock, has already cloned more than 500 dogs. It also plans to revive extinct animals, like the mammoth, in a scenario reminiscent of *Jurassic Park*. In 2021, the American biotech company Colossal, led by Professor George Church of Harvard, initiated a project to create Asian elephant embryos modified by the insertion of mammoth DNA, a transgenesis approach that allows the creation of hybrid animals. The official goal of this project is to produce a breed of cold-resistant animals to populate and preserve the Siberian tundra, and thus help to capture greenhouse gases!

media, duplicating the consciousness, memory, thoughts, knowledge, and emotions of the human brain on a digital medium seems totally implausible today. In parallel, the use of AI and digital technologies is also explored to preserve the memory of the deceased in the form of conversational agents called *deadbots*. These are trained from written or vocal messages exchanged by the person during their lifetime. These *deadbots* can then conduct conversations well beyond simple programmed exchanges, reproducing the thought, reasoning, and even the sense of humor of the deceased.[6]

Fighting against death will not be the only concern of the man of the twenty-first century. Technologies will also be called upon to offer a dignified end of life to the elderly, disabled, those suffering from incurable diseases, or simply those disinterested in life. Attitudes and practices are evolving on this subject, in light of the media coverage of situations that are particularly difficult. If requests for assisted suicide were in the past most often linked to unbearable pain resistant to treatment, they are now more often motivated by the loss of autonomy and dignity. Many countries have established legal frameworks to authorize palliative care, at the risk of potentially accelerating death. In France, the Leonetti-Claeys law of 2016 on end of life allows access to lethal medication under certain conditions, associated with different levels of safety. However, this law frequently encounters obstacles of a medical, ethical, religious, and legal nature in its application.

In this context, the question of euthanasia regularly arises, beyond the need to relieve end-of-life patients. Today, legislation distinguishes passive euthanasia, which relies on palliative care, from active euthanasia, whereby health professionals are authorized to assist a patient at the end of life or suffering from an incurable disease, in pain and without other solutions, to die with dignity. In France, the "end of life" commission of the Economic, Social, and Environmental Council mentioned in 2018 the possibility for a seriously ill person wishing to die to receive an "expressly lethal medication," that is, a prescription specifically intended to cause death and not just to relieve pain. Contemporary medicine uses substances that plunge the patient into a painless unconsciousness, for example, barbiturates associated or not with a neuromuscular paralyzing agent or high-dose morphine.

Switzerland has the most progressive legislation in this field. The Swiss Medical Academy, which is a moral authority on the matter, published guidelines on end-of-life care as early as 1995. These first guidelines prohibited active euthanasia and expressed opposition to assisted suicide, which were not considered medical acts. Since then, these guidelines have been updated, particularly to introduce the possibility of assisted suicide. Since 2018, the existence of an incurable disease or an imminent end of life is no longer required in Switzerland, as long as the patient

[6] N. Bostrom. *Superintelligence*. Dunod, 2014. In 2021, a Canadian computer scientist used a *deadbot* based on GPT-3 to continue "conversing" with a simulation of his deceased partner.

testifies to suffering that he or she considers unbearable. The current law, however, imposes three conditions for resorting to assisted suicide: the patient's discernment, the self-administration of the lethal dose, and the verification that no caregiver has selfish motives.[7] Common requests are related to serious and incurable diseases such as cancers, neurodegenerative, cardiovascular, musculoskeletal, and respiratory diseases, as well as severe depression.

In the future, there is a risk of a drift toward requests for assisted suicide linked solely to old age, a claim supported by nearly 70% of the Swiss population. With the significant aging of the population expected in the twenty-first century everywhere in the world, the mindsets will inevitably move beyond the current accompaniment of dependent people at the end of life. The central debate will concern the individual choice of a medically assisted death to help not only the dying in pain but also those tired of a life they consider too long, whatever their reasons.

New Insights into Aging

Many research teams around the world are working to elucidate the mechanisms of aging in order to develop drugs capable of slowing down this programmed degradation of the body, so long mysterious. In 350 BC, Aristotle wondered about the differences in longevity observed in animals. Contemporary science has revealed that natural selection often favors longevity in larger organisms. For example, the bowhead whale can live nearly 200 years, the Galapagos tortoise about 170 years, and elephants more than 60 years. Within the same species, there are significant variations in the lifespan. Thus, a Texan cat named Reme Puff—despite being fed a shamefully rich diet of bacon and fats!—lived 38 years, well beyond the normal life expectancy for a cat. The Australian dog Bluey died at the respectable age of 29 years, more than double the classic lifespan in dogs. In the human species, the Frenchwoman Jeanne Calment currently holds the official longevity record with 122 years, compared to an average of 71 years of life for humans in general (see Box 11.1).

[7] Swiss Academy of Medical Sciences. *Medical-ethical guidelines. Attitude towards the end of life and death*, 2018. The number of assisted suicides continues to increase in Switzerland due to specific laws in some cantons that require public institutions, such as hospitals or retirement homes, to perform these acts. Associations like Dignitas, Exit and Life Circle generally manage these practices. Some of them specifically request to facilitate the access of elderly people to sodium pentobarbital.

Box 11.1: Jeanne Calment and Other Old-Timers

In the pantheon of venerable old people, Methuselah, a legendary biblical character, is famous for having lived, according to the Old Testament, until the respectable age of 969 years! In the real world, biologists estimate that the maximum lifespan for humans is 120 years, although exceptional cases exist. Jeanne Calment, born on February 21, 1875, and died on August 4, 1997, at the age of 122 years, 5 months, and 14 days, holds the officially documented longevity record.[8]

Despite her respectable age at her death, Jeanne Calment's record will likely be beaten soon. It is estimated that about 400 supercentenarians aged over 110 years are currently alive in the world, with some in perfect health. A valuable lesson learned from these individuals with exceptional longevity is that it is possible to stay healthy throughout one's life. These conclusions are also supported by observations of natural aging in animals. Thus, the turtle named Harriet, reportedly brought back from the Galápagos Islands by Charles Darwin, lived up to 176 years while staying healthy for 175 years!

Biologists have sought to explain the apparent differences in lifespan between individuals of the same species. Studies on simple animals quickly confirmed that genetics play an important role in longevity. Mutations in the *age-1* gene allow the worm *Caenorhabditis elegans* to live up to 190 days, which is 10 times its normal lifespan. In parallel, mutations of the *indy* gene (meaning *I am not dead yet!*) increase the lifespan of the fruit fly by 40 to 80 days. Other genetically modified animals, including flies called *Methuselah* and mice nicknamed *Yoda* (in reference to the old Jedi master from *Star Wars*), have been created in the laboratory, also demonstrating an extended lifespan. In mice, the inhibition of genes coding for growth factors, or conversely the overexpression of genes inducing dwarfism, as well as the drastic reduction of food intake, have extended the lifespan—on average 2 years in normal mice—up to almost 5 years! Collectively, these animal experiments demonstrate the combined role of genetic heritage and nutrition in the lifespan of living beings. Moreover, these studies on genetically modified animals confirm that longevity is compatible with good health until the end of life, corroborating observations made during the natural aging of animals and humans. Importantly, there seems to be no "wall of death," an insurmountable biological limit to living a very long time in good conditions.[9]

---

[8] A Russian study recently questioned the real age of the oldest human at her death, arguing that it was actually her daughter who had usurped her identity. This hypothesis is now rejected.

[9] The existence of such a "wall of death" had been suggested by researchers working on the molecular mechanisms of cell death. They had highlighted what was called the Hayflick limit, a concept stating that a cell cannot divide more than about 50 times before dying.

These recent scientific findings—and those to come—will allow the human species to interfere with the aging process during the twenty-first century. As mentioned earlier, in connection with the continuous progress of medicine and hygiene, the life expectancy at birth in humans has increased by about 3 months per year in developed countries since the middle of the twentieth century. In France, this life expectancy was estimated to be 79.3 years for men and 85.2 years for women in 2022. Another interesting metric for judging healthy aging is the life expectancy without disability for people aged 65 years, which is also regularly increasing. This is currently in France: 10.2 years for men and 11.8 years for women. In light of the opportunities offered by new technologies, the ambition to continue increasing life expectancy by delaying the biological aging that causes diseases now appears quite realistic.[10]

To design truly effective drugs against aging, our knowledge on the subject has long remained very insufficient. However, for about a decade, we have begun to better understand these mechanisms operating at the cellular and molecular level. Some are genetically determined and aim to eliminate aging cells. This programmed cell death, essential for renewing tissues by eliminating cells likely to lose their function or become cancerous, has been selected by natural evolution. The molecular workings that trigger this cell death are better understood, especially those related to the length of telomeres that protect the ends of chromosomes when cells divide.[11] Over successive cell divisions, telomeres shorten until a senescence signal triggers the cell's suicide. Cellular aging mechanisms also involve oxidative metabolism, which damages many molecules such as DNA, lipids, and proteins. Chronic inflammation, somatic mutations, epigenetic alterations, changes in chromatin structure, dysfunction of autophagy, decreased energy production by mitochondria, and decreased metabolic capacities of the cell are also part of these mechanisms. Other alterations of biological processes operate at the organism level. The functional decline of stem cells, the weakening of immune defenses, the increased risk of cancerous transformation, or the accumulation of prions, which are likely to induce neurodegenerative diseases, are all phenomena directly related to aging. In total, contemporary research today points to about a dozen biological processes disturbed in connection with aging that could be targeted by drug approaches.[12]

---

[10] See the Report from the Directorate of Research, Studies, Evaluation, and Statistics on life expectancy in France without disability, December 2023.

[11] Cabon et al. [3]. Different types of cell death have been identified, including necrosis, apoptosis, and autophagy, as well as others that are still poorly understood. Necrosis results from the rupture of the cell membrane, while apoptosis is a programmed process that leads to the fragmentation of DNA in the cell nucleus. Autophagy involves the intracellular digestion of cytoplasmic components. Most cells are equipped with an enzyme called telomerase, whose role is to slow down the loss of telomere length.

[12] Lopez-Otín et al. [4]. Multiple mechanisms of aging of the immune system, called immunosenescence, have been described, affecting all components of immunity. A progressive loss of immune system effectiveness makes older individuals more susceptible to infectious diseases and cancers.

To effectively interfere with natural aging, it is essential to expand current knowledge. In this regard, AI is now widely used to analyze data related to the molecular mechanisms involved in certain rare aging diseases, such as progeria, a genetic disease caused by a recently identified mutation.[13] Children with progeria age rapidly; they look like older people even though they are only a few years old, and most often die of old age before the age of 15. Conversely, a few rare cases have been described worldwide of newborns who do not seem to age or do so very slowly. These children suffer from what is called Benjamin Button's disease, the mechanisms of which are unknown to this day.[14] The fate of these children is not at all enviable, as they show severe developmental disorders and remain unable to walk, talk, or feed themselves, even when they are about 10 years old. Thanks to AI, the data available on these extreme aging anomalies can be exploited in parallel with those obtained by exhaustive molecular profiling of supercentenarians aged 110 and over to understand the biological mechanisms that keep these individuals in top shape. These multidimensional analyses will help to clarify the mechanisms that promote aging or protect against it and thus, identify targets for designing future drugs to inhibit harmful biological processes and stimulate beneficial ones in terms of longevity.

In addition to advances in scientific knowledge that open up new opportunities, we will see later that a major interest in the development of anti-aging drugs is that it could significantly reduce health costs. If aging cannot be completely abolished for fear of causing a catastrophic senescence of humanity, we have already succumbed to the temptation to fight it, sometimes in surprising ways. With the help of AI, of course!

Soon, the First Anti-aging Drugs?

From the above, it comes that some medical advances envisaged by 2050 could slow down the aging process well beyond anti-wrinkle creams, skin lifts, or other cosmetic solutions that improve appearance but do not impact biological age. Healthy aging has emerged as a new discipline to lay the scientific foundations for specialized anti-aging medicine. Concretely, this could combine behavioral changes—in terms of physical activity and nutrition—with innovative treatments previously mentioned, such as tissue regeneration using stem cells, artificial organs, or printed tissues to repair failing body parts. Other approaches, currently

[13] This mutation affects a protein called Lamin A, whose function is to maintain the structure and stability of cell nuclei. In patients with progeria, the mutated gene produces a truncated protein that proves to be toxic.

[14] In reference to the fictional film recounting *The Curious Case of Benjamin Button*, an imaginary character whose biological clock runs backward: born with the appearance of a wrinkled old man, he progressively rejuvenates as time passes until he transforms into an infant.

experimental, consider genetically reprogramming cells from older subjects to give them the functionalities of younger cells.[15]

In the short term, the most relevant approach consists of pharmacological treatments targeting the biological processes involved in aging to prevent the emergence and progression of various diseases. Despite the multiplicity of mechanisms involved, many biotechnology companies have already undertaken to develop drugs to slow down aging. Before discussing the significant contributions of AI in this area, we will mention the anti-aging drug candidates that have given encouraging results in animals and are currently being evaluated in humans. These drug molecules include DHEA, telomerase activators, the antidiabetic metformin, NAD precursors, and antioxidants. Other approaches focus on caloric restriction or rapamycin-based treatments that mimic this effect.[16] However, the drugs that are currently attracting the most interest are GLP-1 analogs, which, as we have seen, are used in the treatment of obesity. Recent results confirm, indeed, that these drugs lower the risk of cardiovascular diseases encompassing heart failure, hypertension, and strokes, as well as certain cancers. The potential benefits of these drugs are currently being evaluated in patients with Alzheimer's disease. It is therefore possible that this therapeutic class, by preventing the occurrence of diseases associated with obesity, may extend both the lifespan and healthy life expectancy.

In parallel, another surprising strategy to fight against aging uses a method dating back 150 years, called parabiosis, with notable support from Peter Thiel, founder of PayPal. Historically, this technique consisted of connecting the blood vessels of two animals so that the blood of a young individual could circulate in the body of an elderly individual to revitalize the latter. Tests on rats have confirmed that exposure to the blood of young specimens—for several months, however!—led to an increase in the lifespan of older subjects compared to control animals. A plausible explanation is that "young" blood contains factors that stimulate stem cells in older animals. In 2015, the Californian company Alkahest tested a similar approach on patients with Alzheimer's disease by regularly administering them plasma from young subjects. Although the results in humans have been disappointing so far, research continues in this field, with a particular interest in the identification of molecules circulating in "young" blood, which would be capable of inducing a rejuvenation in seniors.[17]

---

[15] Several Silicon Valley billionaires, including Jeff Bezos, have invested in companies like Altos Labs and Newlimit, specializing in reprogramming gene expression to prolong human life. In 2022, a British team reported the genetic manipulation in the laboratory of skin cells obtained from a 53-year-old woman to transform them into stem cells capable of producing cells "30 years younger". These latter behave indeed like skin cells of a 20-year-old human in various laboratory tests analyzing their migratory capacity or their contribution to tissue repair.

[16] Dehydroepiandrosterone (DHEA) appears to have anti-aging properties, while nicotinamide adenine dinucleotide (NAD) has shown revitalizing effects in some animal models. Rapamycin, commonly used as an immunosuppressant, is being tested at low doses to mitigate the progressive decline of cardiac and immune functions, frequently observed in elderly people.

[17] Scuderalli [5]. Despite the lack of evidence of effectiveness in humans, some companies in California have undertaken to market repeated transfusions of blood from donors under 25 years old, at a price of $8000 US per liter! This practice was recently suspended by the FDA.

Following the parabiosis experiments, another anti-aging approach being considered involves the use of stem cells, which, due to their progenitor function, constantly divide to give birth to new cells. However, stem cells also show signs of aging over time, consecutively with mutations and epigenetic modifications that reduce their ability to reproduce. One exception is particularly attracting the attention of researchers: that of the stem cells of the jellyfish *Hydra vulgaris*, whose renewal capacity seems preserved over long periods. These creatures indeed show no signs of aging during the observation periods in the laboratory that extend up to 10 years. Understanding the molecular mechanisms underlying this phenomenon could inspire future stem cell-based treatments in humans. In the meantime, wealthy people are opting for the preservation of stem cells present in abundance in the umbilical cord blood of their newborn by freezing these at birth. They thus hope that their offspring will be able to use them for therapeutic purposes in adulthood, if necessary.[18]

How can AI contribute to this field? Its contributions are multiple and could prove decisive. First, AI is currently being used to develop a new class of drugs to specifically eliminate senescent cells. In the short term, AI analysis of data from research on the molecular and cellular mechanisms of aging will undoubtedly identify new original therapeutic targets. Several biotechs are already developing drugs targeting proteins that distinguish aging cells from healthy cells. The goal of this approach is not to achieve eternal youth but rather to prevent the inflammation caused by these dying cells. AI has recently identified interesting targets for designing the first so-called "senolytic" drugs, based on synthetic small chemical molecules or monoclonal antibodies. The Broad Institute in Boston has thus trained artificial neural networks to identify among over 800,000 chemical molecules some drug candidates with promising senolytic properties, which are currently being studied for confirmation. Other approaches rely on stimulating patients' immune cells to recognize these molecules associated with senescence and specifically destroy the cells that carry them in order to eventually create an anti-aging vaccine or immunotherapy.

Beyond this, AI could overcome a major obstacle, hitherto insurmountable, to develop anti-aging drugs: the evaluation of their effectiveness in clinical studies. Indeed, unlike the traditional drug approach, which consists of fighting the effects of a disease on a specific organ or function, to be effective, anti-aging drugs will need to act systemically to prevent age-related alterations in the entire body. The question then arises as to the criteria to use in human studies to demonstrate the effectiveness of such drugs. Should we measure muscle loss, the decrease in bone mass, or the decline in cognitive or immune functions? A treatment that would slow the failure of a specific organ without preserving overall physical and cognitive performance could lead to people who live longer but in a state of dependence.

[18] This approach was recently authorized in Europe, sparking criticism from part of the medical community, on the grounds that it lacks scientific evidence at this stage.

Because the issue of aging is not reduced to the simple lifespan, the quality of life, which encompasses various dimensions of healthy aging, is also a crucial parameter.

Another difficulty related to the evaluation of the effectiveness of anti-aging drug candidates is that it requires clinical studies on large cohorts of individuals followed for decades. Until recently, demonstrating the ability of a drug to slow aging seemed out of reach for ages, given this very long evaluation of its effectiveness and safety in humans. AI could, in this indication, allow for the simulation—in accelerated mode—of large, very long-term studies with hundreds of thousands of virtual patients. These virtual patients can be realistically modeled by exploiting, thanks to AI, the medical records accumulated during the follow-up over time of many individuals belonging to different age groups, reflecting the heterogeneity within the human species in the face of healthy aging for some, punctuated by diseases for others. The performance of drug candidates predicted by these models provided by AI could then be corroborated by verifying that the predictions on virtual patients are consistent with the first observations collected during the administration of future drugs to real patients.

The twenty-first century could therefore see the emergence of drugs that prolong healthy life, in parallel with a significant improvement in treatments against chronic diseases, allowing patients who suffer from them to live almost normally. There were only 23,000 centenarians in the world in 1950, and there were 500,000 in 2020. The United Nations Population Fund estimates that there could be 3.2 million in 2050! This anticipated accelerated aging of the human population will have immediate consequences on end-of-life care management, with an expected explosion of dependency. More generally, it will constitute one of the many societal challenges and issues that will need to be addressed during the century.

References

1. Alexandre L. La mort de la mort. Paris: J.-C. Lattes; 2011.
2. Oldak B, et al. Complete human day 14 post-implantation embryo models from naïve ES cells. Nature. 2023;622:567.
3. Cabon L, et al. La mort cellulaire programmée ne manque pas de vocabulaire. Med Sci. 2013;29:1117.
4. Lopez-Otín C, et al. Hallmarks of aging: an expanding universe. Cell. 2023;186:243.
5. Scuderalli M. Blood to blood. Nature. 2015;517:426.

Part IV

New Challenges for Society

A Restructuring of Health Systems

12

How Much Does an Innovative Drug Cost?

It is already well recognized that the health systems of developed countries will have to be deeply rethought to cope with the increase in costs associated with population aging. To measure the magnitude of the task, let's specify that this awareness does not take yet into account the wave of innovative drugs they will face in the coming decades, thanks to AI.

To understand this issue in more detail, let's first examine the mechanisms that determine today's costs and prices of drugs. While regulation has the advantage of establishing the standards for the development and evaluation of drugs, it makes this process particularly long and expensive. On average, the development of a drug takes 12 years and costs USD 2.6 billion to pharmaceutical companies. This exorbitant amount is explained because it includes not only the research and development expenses related to the drug put on the market, but also those associated with all the drug candidates abandoned during development, that is, 93% of the molecules tested![1] These costs and delays have been in constant increase in recent decades, in parallel with a decrease in the success rate of new drug development. Bringing a new drug to the market is complex for several reasons. On the one hand, regulatory authorities require more and more data from animal and human studies, which adds to the burden of industry. In addition, throughout the stages of drug development, there is a significant attrition of projects due to unsatisfactory results. These failures, especially during human clinical trials, are particularly costly. As a result, the

[1] DiMasi et al. [1]. While the development of a drug takes on average 12 years from conception to registration, some drugs take much longer to develop. A case in point is the development of Mosquirix®, the first vaccine against malaria, which spanned over 30 years! Conversely, in exceptional emergency situations, other drugs have been developed in 1 or 2 years, such as for example the vaccines against COVID-19, or gene therapies against rare and severe genetic diseases.

P. Moingeon, *Intelligent Drugs: How AI is Transforming Healthcare*, https://doi.org/10.1007/978-3-031-91668-7_12

efficiency of investment to bring a new drug to the market has halved every 9 years, a trend ironically nicknamed "Eroom's law," as it is the reverse of Moore's law!

Pending the benefits of the revolution induced by AI, pharmaceutical companies currently pass on the costs related to the complexity of development to the prices of drugs. With, as a consequence, often high prices for innovative drugs and sometimes prohibitive treatment costs for chronic diseases that require lifelong treatment. We have mentioned the major progress in recent years in the treatment of cancers, immune-inflammatory diseases, and infectious diseases, thanks to new biological or chemical drugs. Some of these drugs have the status of blockbusters, that is, they generate annual revenues on the scale of billions of US dollars for the laboratories that developed them. For example, Pfizer's Prevnar® vaccine against pneumococcal infections generated annual revenues of nearly USD 6 billion, and AbbVie's anti-TNFα Humira® for treating immune-inflammatory diseases generated revenues of nearly USD 20 billion.[2] The annual sales prospects of the new blockbuster from Sanofi, Dupixent®, an antibody that neutralizes the activity of inflammatory cytokines in atopic dermatitis, are estimated at USD 10 billion. These significant figures must be put into perspective with the societal benefit offered, namely major improvements in the treatment of severe diseases that benefit millions of patients, but also health systems avoiding considerable hospital costs.

For two decades, this traditional model of blockbuster drugs at controlled prices, intended for large patient populations, has gradually been disappearing.[3] With the evolution toward precision medicine, it is now common to see drugs marketed to treat small groups of patients. This new economic model, based on niche busters and adopted by pharmaceutical companies, relies on lower sales volumes but higher prices based on a substantial therapeutic improvement for a defined subgroup of patients.

As a result, an increasing number of drugs brought to the market that revolutionize the management of certain diseases result in annual treatment costs per patient ranging from tens of thousands to millions of US dollars (see Table 12.1). In particular, in recent years, several gene therapies, including Zolgensma®, Hemgenix®, and Lenmeldy®, have been made available to patients to treat rare genetic diseases,

---

[2] The sales figures given are those of 2017. The Prevnar® vaccine effectively protects young children and adults against diseases (otitis, meningitis, respiratory tract infections) caused by the bacterium *Streptococcus pneumoniae*. Humira® has revolutionized the treatment of chronic inflammatory diseases such as rheumatoid arthritis, psoriasis, Crohn's disease, and ulcerative colitis.

[3] This evolution has resulted in a significant reduction in the return on investment in research and development for the pharmaceutical industry. Source: *Deloitte Centre for Health solutions and Global Data. Unlocking R and D productivity: measuring the return from pharmaceutical innovation*, 2018. With an average development cost of $2.6 billion US, a new drug now generates an average of estimated maximum annual sales of $400 million US. To be compared respectively with the figures in 2010 of $1.2 billion US in development cost associated with $800 million US in annual sales.

Table 12.1 Selection of some of the most expensive drugs

Drug (laboratory)	Indications	Cost per patient per year	Therapeutic contribution
Gilenya® (Novartis)	Multiple sclerosis	USD 48,000	Launched in 2010, this first oral treatment for multiple sclerosis was, at the time, the most expensive for this autoimmune disease. It is now the cheapest! It reduces the relapse rate by half in the relapsing form but fails to slow down the disease in its progressive form
Sovaldi® (Gilead)	Hepatitis C	Total treatment cost of €56,000	This drug is a breakthrough innovation, as it cures 90% of patients with hepatitis C by completely eliminating the virus in 12 weeks of treatment. By the end of 2016, competing drugs, such as Zepatier® (Merck) and Harvoni® (Gilead), were introduced, with a cost of €29,000 for a 3-month treatment
Keytruda® (Merck), Yervoy® and Opdivo® (Bristol Myers Squibb), and Perjeta®, Kadcyla®, and Tecentriq® (Roche)	Metastatic melanoma, breast, lung, ENT, kidney, bladder cancers, Hodgkin's disease, lymphomas	USD 40,000 to 125,000	These different immune checkpoint inhibitors are treatments against various cancers that have an innovative mechanism of action. They lift the inhibition of the immune system frequently observed in patients with cancer, thus reactivating an anti-tumor immune response. These antibody-based drugs have dramatically improved the treatment of blood cancers and are now actively tested in solid tumors in combination with different chemotherapies
Spinraza® (Biogen)	Spinal muscular atrophy linked to the SMN1 gene	€420,000 the first year, half less in the following years.	The first drug against proximal spinal muscular atrophy, Spinraza® (nusinersen), is an antisense oligonucleotide that increases the production of the SMN protein essential for the survival of motor neurons
Glybera® (UniQure)	Rare genetic deficiency in lipoprotein lipase (about 3500 patients worldwide)	Over a million euros	This first gene therapy brought to the market in Europe in 2012 was a commercial failure, as only one patient was treated, who did not need to be treated afterward

(continued)

Table 12.1 (continued)

Drug (laboratory)	Indications	Cost per patient per year	Therapeutic contribution
Zolgensma® (Novartis)	Spinal muscular atrophy	€1.9 million in a single dose	This gene therapy is applied to the treatment of children under 2 years old at the early or pre-symptomatic stage of their disease. The remarkable effectiveness of the treatment in slowing down or preventing the progression of the disease was confirmed after a 5-year follow-up
Hemgenix® (CSL Behring)	Type B hemophilia (congenital deficiency in coagulation factor IX)	USD 3.5 million	This gene therapy (etranacogene dezaparvovec) developed by UniQure is based on an adeno-associated viral vector expressing the gene of factor IX; it only requires a single administration
Lenmeldy® (orchard therapeutics)	Metachromatic Leukodystrophy	USD 4.25 million	In March 2024, this gene therapy based on a retroviral vector became the most expensive drug in the world as a single-dose treatment for an ultra-rare neurological disease associated with a loss of motor skills

at a cost of several million US dollars. Fortunately, it requires only one administration.

According to some estimates, in the next 5 years, hundreds of gene therapy drugs could be registered to treat diseases such as blood diseases, certain forms of blindness, and rare neurodegenerative or muscular conditions. Beyond that, nearly 1800 gene therapy treatments are currently under development, of which 25% target neurological disorders. With an average cost estimated at USD one million per year for treating a single patient, this wave of innovative drugs will have a significant impact on the budgets of health systems. This level of pricing is currently justified by the fact that these treatments radically transform the prognosis of the disease, with a possible cure after a single injection for patients who, in most cases, have no therapeutic alternative.[4]

We have seen that AI now allows health industry professionals to make much better decisions when designing and developing new drugs. We can therefore expect

[4] Moreover, these treatments are aimed at rare diseases, a high price is thus the consequence of reduced sales volumes, in order to allow the manufacturer to recoup its development investments.

that the chances of success in future developments will increase significantly, resulting in a reduction in the costs and time required to make a new drug available to patients. Most likely, the synergies between AI and drug sciences will pave the way, in the coming decades, for the arrival on the market of many breakthrough intelligent drugs, some of which are potentially very expensive. In the face of these recent and upcoming developments, it will be essential to market these innovative drugs at an acceptable price so that they can be covered by health systems.

More Drugs for Less, with AI

The issue of a fair price for drugs is crucial. However, this is a complex challenge, involving, from a societal point of view, ensuring access to treatments for all patients while ensuring the budgetary balance of care systems. At the same time, a fair reward for innovation is an essential condition to attract the private investments necessary for the development of innovative drugs. The price of a drug cannot, therefore, simply be based on production costs or raw materials to make a tablet, as one might naively think. From the drug industry's point of view, it is obviously necessary to take into account the expenses incurred for all developments, including those that have failed. Added to this are the costs related to production and distribution infrastructures, which are often significant, especially for biological drugs.[5]

Unlike a consumer product, the price of a drug is not left solely to the choice of the manufacturer. Today, the setting of the price and the conditions for reimbursement of the drug are subject to specific regulations, varying by country, in the absence of uniform international standards. However, a widely established consensus in developed countries is that the price of a drug should be linked to its societal utility, with a *value-based pricing* indexed on the therapeutic benefit brought to patients. In the United States, the price of a new drug is free; however, price and reimbursement are eventually decided during negotiations reflecting the interests of manufacturers and payers, the latter bringing together public or private health insurance funds.[6]

The specific case of determining the price and reimbursement of drugs in France, used here as a representative of the tightly regulated European approach, is discussed in Box 12.1.

[5]The introduction of a new drug on the market requires considerable investments in the development of manufacturing methods, production facilities, and the establishment of a distribution chain. More than half of the major therapeutic advances currently come from biological products, whose development is costly. The complexity of the production processes and characterization of these biological drugs indeed results in higher costs than for drugs based on small chemical molecules.

[6]The United States commonly accounts for 30% of global sales, but with significant discounts imposed on manufacturers by private health insurance, which have a strong bargaining power to grant their reimbursement.

Box 12.1: Price and Reimbursement of Drugs in France

The price of the drug is regulated for all drugs that are reimbursed by Social Security.[7] In its determination, the first step consists of the evaluation of the therapeutic efficacy of the new drug compared to any existing treatments in order to decide on its societal interest in terms of cost-benefit. To this end, the High Authority for Health (HAS) evaluates the medical service provided by the new drug. The price is then set by the Economic Committee for Health Products on this basis, taking also into account the potential existence of comparator drugs already on the market. The Ministry of Health then determines the reimbursement rate of the drug, which can range from 0% to 100% of its price, depending on the case.[8]

The initial assessment of the performance of the drug is based on clinical trials, but scientific knowledge evolves during its real-life use, leading to periodic reassessments of the conditions of coverage. For example, some drugs against Alzheimer's disease have seen their rating go from "important" to "low" and then "insufficient" over the years, leading to a progressive decrease in their reimbursement.[9]

After setting the initial marketing price of a drug, this evolves over time in response to several regulatory mechanisms, briefly mentioned here. Firstly, market mechanisms—the famous "invisible hand" theorized by Adam Smith—constitute a powerful downward regulator of drug prices after their market launch. These mechanisms rely on competition between pharmaceutical companies, encouraged by governments and public regulatory agencies. An innovative drug does not remain long alone on the market for a given indication, with most often rapidly registered competing products that form a new therapeutic class intended to treat a given disease.[10]

[7] It is free and can be unilaterally set by the laboratory only for non-reimbursable drugs.

[8] The HAS is a public authority of a scientific nature (www.has-sante.fr). The medical service rendered takes into account the severity of the disease as well as various data specific to the drug (efficacy, side effects, existence of therapeutic alternatives, interest for public health) in a particular indication.

[9] The administered prices of drugs in France are among the lowest in Europe: 40% cheaper than in Switzerland, 33% cheaper than in Germany and 18% cheaper than in Italy. As a result, the drug market in France is not always considered attractive by pharmaceutical companies, which partly explains the shortages of an increasing number of drugs in this country.

[10] As an example, the rapid registration of several drugs competing with Solvadi® quickly halved the price of the treatment for hepatitis C (see Table 12.1).

Another price regulation mechanism consists of the marketing of generics and biosimilars, copies of original drugs marketed at significantly lower prices, when patents have expired. Generics refer to copies of drugs based on chemical molecules, while biosimilars are copies of biological drugs, for example, monoclonal antibodies. It should be noted that biological products are more difficult to copy due to their complex molecular composition.[11] Moreover, large pharmaceutical companies practice tier pricing, a system consisting of marketing drugs at a significantly lower price in low-income countries compared to developed countries. Gilead Sciences has thus marketed Solvadi® in Egypt (the country most affected in the world by the hepatitis C virus) at prices 100 times lower than those practiced in developed countries.

To cope with the revolution of intelligent drugs, international coordination to regulate prices appears highly desirable. However, it is unlikely that this will happen in the short term, due to the very different health insurance systems depending on the country. Nonetheless, there is a common will to adapt prices over time that revolves around the paradigm of pay-for-performance, that is, the idea that prices and reimbursements of drugs should be indexed on their actual performance after marketing.[12] This approach has the advantage of focusing the resources of health systems on drugs that provide a significant therapeutic benefit. A difficulty to overcome, however, is the assessment of the performance of drugs when they are used on a large scale. On this subject, we have seen the significant contribution of AI to analyze the data on the efficacy and safety of new drugs generated after their market launch. The level of coverage initially established at the time of drug registration can thus be confirmed—or adjusted—based on extremely precise performance metrics, documented in real life, thanks to AI. Beyond this, the progressive deployment of predictive models based on AI and their regulatory acceptability may allow in the long term for a fair determination of the selling price and the reimbursement rate, moving from a system of pay-for-performance toward an approach of pay-for-predicted-performance.

---

[11] A patent grants a monopoly of exploitation to its owner for about 20 years, allowing him to recoup his investments in innovation. When the patent that protects the original drug (called *princeps*) expires, sales can quickly drop by more than 90% upon the introduction of competing generics.

[12] In France, since 2014, the pharmaceutical industry and the health authorities have established performance contracts to adjust drug prices, particularly anticancer drugs, based on their actual effectiveness. The United Kingdom uses the QALY (*quality-adjusted life year*, year of life gained in good health) to evaluate new costly therapies. The *National Institute for Health and Clinical Excellence* (NICE) in the UK has set at €35,000 the acceptable cost for the health system for an additional year of life gained through a new anticancer treatment. Similarly, the Netherlands reimburses anticancer treatments up to €80,000 per year of life gained in good health. However, this accounting approach has been criticized as it may favor patients deemed socially useful and, conversely, restrict access to expensive drugs for end-of-life patients.

In the context of health budget constraints, a major benefit of AI is that it will gradually—and significantly—reduce the development costs of new drugs. The continuous increase observed over the last 20 years in the average development cost is no longer sustainable. However, AI not only accelerates discovery but will also benefit the development of new innovative drugs by improving the chances of success during clinical trials, thanks to the upstream design of a better drug candidate. Furthermore, the increasing use of virtual patients will significantly reduce the expenses associated with clinical studies by reducing their size and duration. The prospect of substantial savings in development costs for the drug industry should result in the marketing of future drugs at reasonable prices. If not, the revolution of intelligent drugs will result in an influx of innovative treatments that will inevitably overwhelm the capacities of existing health systems.

Horizon 2050: How to Distribute the Value Created by AI in Health?

In the coming decades, the revolution of intelligent drugs will require solving a real squaring of the circle: balancing the cost of incentivizing drug innovation with that of its societal coverage. While it is clear that AI will generate a lot of value in the health field, it remains to be defined how this will be shared among the different stakeholders, namely patients, health professionals, the drug industry, and payers.

By 2050, patients will very likely be the big winners of the ongoing revolution, with drugs that are more effective, safer, and better suited to their needs and specificities. Continuous progress—often spectacular—will be made in the treatment of diseases currently without a therapeutic option or poorly managed. Following the advances of recent years, it will become possible to live with most chronic diseases, controlled with the help of drugs—alone or in combination—well tolerated. New treatments for cancers currently poorly treated, affecting, for example, the lung, the pancreas, the stomach, or the brain, will significantly increase the life expectancy of patients. Drugs will be developed to treat—or slow down—most neurodegenerative diseases and those related to aging. Precision medicine will become increasingly personalized, and a growing number of rare diseases will be effectively managed. Sophisticated models of each patient's disease, in the form of a digital twin, virtual patient, or even a digital avatar, will allow the evaluation of a multitude of treatments to select the most appropriate one. Another positive evolution for patients will be the opportunity for them to engage more in the management of their health.

The provision of intelligent drugs will also benefit health professionals by offering them more and more treatment options, more effective and better tolerated, for their patients, as well as new possibilities for early screening and diagnosis, decision support, and telemedicine enhanced by more immersive virtual reality. The applications of AI combined with the deployment of digital tools should hopefully allow health professionals to reduce their administrative tasks so that they can focus more on medical and scientific activities. This evolution will, however, require a necessary acculturation to these new technologies so that they are perceived and used as complementary tools to their expertise and not as a substitute.

For the health industry, the value created by AI will also be very important, with, as we have seen, an acceleration already perceptible in the discovery of new drugs. As we progress in this century, the pharmaceutical industry will carry out an increasing part of the activities necessary for the design, preclinical development, and evaluation of the performance of any new drug by computer. Only a small number of drug molecules selected with predictive models will then be produced to be tested in clinical studies with real patients, in parallel with virtual models. The cost and duration of developing a new drug will be significantly reduced, with the probability of success considerably increased. In return for these benefits, the pharmaceutical industry will have to agree on reasonable prices for these intelligent drugs, ensuring its profitability by marketing them in larger numbers.

It is clear that for the health systems of developed countries, whether they are public or private insurance, the challenges will be the most significant in order to control costs in the context of drug innovation fueled by AI. In France, total health expenditures amounted to nearly €314 billion in 2022. The expenditures specifically related to drugs were nearly €33 billion, compared to 115 and 121 billion for the costs associated with hospital care and outpatient care, respectively. Globally, drug expenditures are estimated at USD 1500 billion and could reach USD 2000 billion by 2027, an annual growth rate of 4.6%.[13] The increase in drug-related expenditures is due to three well-identified factors. First, an increase in the price of drugs, which in this case should not be significant by 2050 if the contributions of AI are reflected by a decrease in prices by the pharmaceutical industry. The second factor is that of population growth and aging. This aging is associated with an estimated 3% annual increase in the number of people suffering from chronic diseases or in a state of dependence.[14] The third factor increasing expenses is the rising abundance of innovative drugs. In just the last 5 years, over 70 new cancer treatments have been developed, improving the quality of life of millions of patients and the prognosis of more than 20 different types of cancers. In light of AI, but also of biotechnologies and gene therapy, the supply of new drugs could be plentiful by 2050.

---

[13] See the DREES (Directorate for Research, Studies, Evaluation, and Statistics) report for France: *Résultats des comptes de la santé: Édition 2023*. International health expenditures include the consumption of care and medical goods (hospital care, outpatient and city care, drugs) and expenditures related to long-term care, prevention, and health system governance. For global figures, see the report *IQVIA Global use of medicine 2023*.

[14] To illustrate the magnitude and speed of the expected aging of the population, it is estimated that, among people born in the 1980s, half of the men and two-thirds of the women will reach the age of 90. Half of the children born after 2000 could become centenarians or supercentenarians! The favorable impact of AI on the emergence of new effective drugs, some of which could potentially act on aging, will only accelerate this demographic evolution. The question will arise of the cost for health systems of these aging people, and more particularly of the management in developed countries of a "fourth age" sociologically defined as people over 75 who have become dependent. Or even a "fifth age" gathering seniors well over 100 years old!

These developments raise the specific issue of the distribution of resources allocated to the health system among patients, depending on the diseases they suffer from. Concretely, the management of chronic diseases, which, in France, affects less than 20% of patients, today represents 80% of health costs.[15] This challenge is now taking a particular turn with the development of an increasing number of high-tech drugs intended for patients suffering from rare diseases, also called orphan diseases. These diseases, numbering around 7000, are often very serious, have a genetic cause for more than 70% of them, and manifest from early childhood. As their name suggests, each of these rare diseases affects a small number of patients, for example, a few dozen to a few tens of thousands worldwide. Yet, collectively, these conditions affect more than 300 million people, or nearly 4% of the world population![16] AI coupled with DNA and RNA targeting methods should, in the coming years, allow for the design of effective treatments for an increasing number of these rare diseases. It will therefore be imperative to find new solutions so that health systems can take charge of these future drugs to help patients suffering from such diseases while preserving the budgetary balance of health systems based on solidarity.

Part of the answer to the problem must come from new technologies. AI and digital technologies can contribute to savings by facilitating the dematerialized exchange of health data, the development of telemedicine, the digital transformation of hospitals, and the efficient management of patients.[17] In parallel, the acceleration by AI of a transition toward preventive medicine could be a source of substantial savings for health systems. On the pharmacoeconomic level, recent studies suggest that for USD 1000 spent today by developed countries on health, only USD 1 is invested in prevention! The implementation of a medicine more based on preventive

[15] More than ten million people, or 17% of the population, are currently fully covered by Social Security for a long-term illness, such as cardiovascular diseases, cancers, metabolic diseases (especially diabetes, which alone accounts for 15% of expenditures), respiratory diseases, or Alzheimer's disease. These are most often elderly people, i.e., two-thirds of men and half of women over 75.

[16] The Orphanet database, coordinated by INSERM in France, gathers detailed epidemiological data on these rare diseases worldwide. For the majority of them, there was no effective treatment before the emergence of gene therapy or oligonucleotide-based treatments. To improve the treatments of these diseases, a challenge is to develop a concerted international health policy, focusing on specific priorities. About 150 of them are responsible for 80% of rare disease cases. In many developed countries, governments encourage companies to develop drugs in these indications, for example by granting a period of commercial exclusivity protecting from competition.

[17] Before the COVID-19 crisis, France aimed to limit the annual increase in its health expenditures between 2% and 3%. To do this, the country has focused its efforts in recent years on reducing drug consumption, restructuring hospitals, consolidating health services, developing outpatient surgery, reducing medical transport costs, eliminating unnecessary prescriptions, and using generic drugs. More recently, the solutions considered are to increase the medical deductible, i.e., the amount remaining to be paid by patients for drug boxes or doctor consultations, as well as to raise awareness among doctors and patients of the need for sobriety in drug consumption. Internationally, the OECD has also encouraged the reduction of hospital costs, favoring home care and the use of telemedicine to limit visits to emergency departments.

drugs—and no longer curative—represents a serious path to achieve considerable savings in health costs. As an example, drugs capable of delaying aging by only 1 year—and thus preventing many age-related diseases—could, according to some estimates, lead to health cost savings reaching up to USD 37 trillion for the United States alone [2, 3]!

References

1. DiMasi JA, et al. Innovation in the pharmaceutical industry: new estimates of R&D costs. J Health Econ. 2016;47:20.
2. Steele A. Ageless: the new science of getting older without getting old. *Bloomsbury Editor, 2022.*
3. Scott A, et al. The economic value of targeting aging. Nat Aging. 2021;1:616.

13 Restoring Trust in Drugs

Better Manage the Side Effects

Despite their major contribution to the treatment of many diseases, public opinion remains ambivalent toward drugs. How, for example, can we explain the rejection by part of the population of COVID-19 vaccines, which, according to the WHO, have saved the lives of 20 million people in 2021 alone? The first answer lies in the proliferation of information, disseminated through social networks and traditional media, questioning the effectiveness of certain drugs, even when it is scientifically documented. Misinformation also concerns side effects, arguing that these are minimized by health authorities and the pharmaceutical industry. While these unwanted effects are most often limited and/or restricted to a fraction of the population, their scope is amplified by rumors to feed a mistrust of the general public—and sometimes even health professionals—toward drugs. Before the COVID-19 crisis, distrust toward pharmaceutical companies was particularly prevalent in the French population. According to a survey by the Odoxa Institute, only 34% of French people had a good opinion of the pharmaceutical industry, whereas 74% of Britons, 67% of Germans, and 69% of Italians trusted them.[1]

A second explanation is the societal unacceptability of the adverse effects of drugs, even moderate ones. This risk aversion is increasingly pronounced in our postmodern society, which is quick to hide behind the famous precautionary principle. As an anecdote, the marketing of a drug such as aspirin—first marketed by Bayer Laboratories in 1899—would not be simple today. Aspirin induces small bleeding, generally imperceptible and not problematic, in the nose, gums, or digestive tract. In very rare cases, for example, from overdose

[1] Digital giants have little control over the veracity of the information disseminated on their platforms. Some media in search of audience are inclined to maintain controversies and radicalize opinions. In France, the Academies of Medicine and of Pharmacy have raised alarms about this misinformation, which raises inappropriate doubts about the effectiveness of drugs.

P. Moingeon, *Intelligent Drugs: How AI is Transforming Healthcare*,
https://doi.org/10.1007/978-3-031-91668-7_13

poisoning or intolerance in certain patients, the side effects can be much more serious. However, the very satisfactory safety profile of aspirin has been confirmed by billions of patients who have used it not only to relieve minor fevers or pains but also to reduce the risk of stroke.

From this example, we note that, due to their mechanism of action, which involves an interaction with a biological process, all drugs are likely to induce adverse effects, especially if they are used at an inadequate dose or in inappropriate patients. In this context, to respond to erroneous messages and often unfounded fears, it is important to communicate transparently and factually about the real side effects of drugs. It is also necessary to inform about the methods used to evaluate the benefit-to-risk ratio of any new drug. We have seen that the benefits of the drug are measured objectively by observing the improvement in the condition of patients treated during clinical trials and then in real-life conditions. Similarly, drug safety is subject to rigorous and regulated monitoring during clinical trials and after marketing. Risks are assessed in terms of adverse reactions in the general population, taking into account their probability and their severity, as well as the possible susceptibilities of certain patients.

Outside their normal use, adverse effects sometimes occur following accidents or even health scandals consequent to the misuse of drugs. These last decades have been marked by several crises related to drugs such as Distilbene® (synthetic estrogen), Isomeride® and Mediator® (appetite suppressant drugs), Cerivastatin® (cholesterol-lowering), Vioxx® (anti-inflammatory), Depakine® (anti-epileptic), certain contraceptive pills, and opioid drugs, including notably Fentanyl®.[2] These drug crises, due to various causes, have negatively affected the opinion on drugs, manufacturers, and sometimes even the health professionals who administered them. In the vast majority of cases, health actors involved in the development, regulatory approval, evaluation, and prescription of the drugs in question have acted in compliance with the regulations, good practices, and scientific knowledge of the time. Sometimes, these serious side effects were only revealed in certain patients during large-scale use, whereas they had not been detected during clinical trials involving a few hundred or thousand patients.

These dramatic situations have led to notable improvements in drug safety surveillance, particularly since the 2000s. We have seen that in-depth studies of

[2] Distilbène®, prescribed in the 1970s to prevent miscarriages in pregnant women, caused vaginal cancers, genital malformations, and infertility in daughters born to treated mothers. Isomeride®@, used as an appetite suppressant, increased the risk of pulmonary arterial hypertension and thickening of the heart valves and was withdrawn in 1997. The Mediator®, originally a treatment for overweight diabetics, was also prescribed as an appetite suppressant, presenting similar effects to Isomeride®, and withdrawn from the market in 2009. Cerivastatin®, withdrawn in 2001, was administered to prevent cardiovascular diseases, causing muscle toxicity in some patients. Vioxx®, used as an anti-inflammatory, caused heart problems in patients treated for more than 18 months, and was withdrawn in 2004. Depakine®, an anti-epileptic drug, caused fetal anomalies in pregnant women and this risk is now specified in the notice. In 2012, third and fourth generation contraceptive pills (so named according to the nature of the progestin entering their composition) were associated with an increased risk of severe thrombosis in women. An opioid crisis has erupted in recent years in the United States due to the prescription and abuse of these painkillers, causing many addictions and many deaths from consumption of excessive doses.

toxicology on animals are now a crucial step in the preclinical evaluation of any new drug. The documentation of side effects and their acceptability in view of the therapeutic benefit are the most important criteria used to authorize—or not—their marketing. In this evaluation, expertise in drug safety and toxicology has been strengthened following health crises, also guaranteeing the independence of the experts consulted, as well as of regulatory agencies and health professionals from pharmaceutical companies. During clinical trials, any serious side effect is now examined by a committee of scientific and medical experts independent of the pharmaceutical laboratory, which has the authority to interrupt the study if necessary.[3]

Pharmacovigilance monitoring has been significantly strengthened throughout the duration of the drug's marketing. In addition to the industry and regulatory experts, health professionals, such as doctors and pharmacists, as well as patients, contribute to the reporting of adverse effects. These data are now collected and shared internationally thanks to digital technologies. AI, as we have seen, will allow us to significantly strengthen drug safety in multiple ways, especially by detecting weak warning signals within vast amounts of data coming from the real-life use of drugs, especially in exchanges between patients on social networks.

Fighting Against Vaccine Hesitancy

A particular form of mistrust toward drugs concerns what is called vaccine hesitancy. This term refers to the growing rejection of vaccines observed in recent years in many developed countries, despite their well-established medical and socio-economic benefits. Numerous studies involving hundreds of billions of administered doses have demonstrated the notable effectiveness of vaccines against many infectious diseases. The vaccine approach consists of administering killed or attenuated viruses or bacteria, or molecules isolated from these infectious agents in order to stimulate a protective immune response without causing real symptoms. This immunity, acquired thanks to the vaccine, will protect the vaccinated individual when they are exposed to these infectious agents in the natural environment. Depending on the case, the immune response induced by the vaccine will prevent infection or attenuate it by protecting against severe forms.

Thanks to vaccination, smallpox has been eradicated, and polio is on its way to being so. On a global scale, mass vaccination has saved billions of lives since Pasteur's work. Vaccines are generally well tolerated, although, like any medication, they can cause adverse effects in a few individuals. Beyond their medical interest due to a risk-benefit ratio that is most often very favorable, the economic value of vaccines is considerable, particularly in developing countries. The total cost to vaccinate a child with the 11 vaccines recommended by the WHO is currently about €50. According to the *Copenhagen Consensus Center*, every euro invested in vaccination campaigns in developing countries generates about €18 in return on

[3] Notably, this committee analyzes whether side effects occur in the group taking the drug or the placebo, and if there is a correlation with the dose.

investment in economic and social terms.[4] In 2016, an international study on population adherence to vaccination (the *Vaccine Confidence Project*) involving 65,000 people in 67 countries showed recognition of the value of vaccines among two-thirds of those surveyed. Since then, distrust has been steadily gaining ground in developed countries in Europe and the USA.[5]

These anti-vaccine individuals, whose numbers are increasing, include not only ultra-religious individuals or those living in rural areas but also city dwellers aspiring to a more natural lifestyle, as well as citizens who do not trust institutions and authorities. In the United States, two out of three people now refuse to be vaccinated against the flu or papillomaviruses. This resistance, although difficult to understand, probably and ironically stems from the success of vaccines in preventing many diseases, thus making the risks associated with these infectious diseases less perceptible to the general public. In the context of the near-total eradication of polio, diphtheria, and tetanus in developed countries, the benefits of these vaccines are no longer visible, and the rare side effects are considered unacceptable.

In discussing the rejection of COVID-19 vaccines, we referred to the desire of some to be able to freely choose whether or not to be vaccinated. However, if vaccination is the most effective tool against infectious diseases, it cannot rely solely on an individual decision but is part of a collective responsibility to also protect others. During an epidemic, it is indeed essential that a high percentage of the population be immunized, either by vaccination or by natural exposure, to halt the spread of the infectious agent. In the context of the SARS-CoV-2 pandemic, it is estimated that at least 80% of the population needs to be immunized to achieve the herd immunity necessary to stop the virus.[6]

In comparison, the spread of measles, which is particularly contagious, requires that 95% of the population be vaccinated. Currently, the global measles vaccination coverage rate is only 85%, which is regularly decreasing in many developed countries. As a result, fatal cases of measles are increasing, mainly among the unvaccinated, with 150,000 people now dying each year from measles, a disease that could be controlled with adequate vaccination coverage.[7] Distrust of the COVID-19 vaccines or measles vaccines is not isolated. The combined pediatric vaccine against measles, mumps, and rubella (MMR) also sparked rejection after cases of autism were observed in a study conducted in the UK in 1998 by Andrew Wakefield on a

---

[4] Vaccines are usually administered by subcutaneous or intramuscular injection, sometimes orally or intranasally. Adverse effects are most often limited to pain at the injection site or a slight fever.

[5] In this study prior to the COVID-19 pandemic, about 70% of French people had confidence in vaccines. Half thought that the benefits of vaccination outweighed the risks, 33% thought they were balanced, and 15% believed that the risks predominated. In addition, 8% considered that child vaccination was not important, 17% doubted the safety of vaccines, and 11% questioned their effectiveness. Today, nearly 8% of American parents request vaccination exemptions for their children, for religious or philosophical reasons.

[6] This percentage of the immunized population includes individuals who have developed protective immunity after being vaccinated against SARS-CoV-2, or infected by the virus.

[7] Schools reserved for unvaccinated children have appeared in the Netherlands and the United States. It is in such establishments that measles or polio outbreaks periodically occur.

dozen patients! Anti-vaccine movements continue to refer to this study, which turned out to be a scientific fraud and whose results have since been refuted by numerous epidemiological studies involving millions of children.[8]

Another important example concerns vaccines against cancer-related viruses. In France, the hepatitis B vaccine was accused of causing multiple sclerosis, an autoimmune disease affecting the nervous system. The link between the vaccine and multiple sclerosis has been refuted by several epidemiological studies, while at the same time, it has been established that this vaccine prevents many liver cancers caused by the hepatitis B virus. Similarly, since 2007, the use of vaccines against oncogenic papillomaviruses to immunize young girls before their sexual activity has reduced the incidence of cervical cancer by more than 90%. Despite its proven effectiveness in millions of girls, a portion of the population still rejects this vaccine, which could eradicate this cancer, the fourth most common cancer in women, killing more than 300,000 women worldwide each year [1].

The WHO has now included this phenomenon of vaccine hesitancy in the top ten major threats to human health, on the grounds that this rejection, based on the ignorance of a minority, compromises protection by herd immunity, thus endangering millions of people. In response to this worrying situation, many developed countries have, rightly, strengthened vaccination obligations in their public health policies. In France, a mandatory program of vaccination for young children against 11 diseases was thus put in place in 2018, without any notable increase in side effects being observed. These vaccines offer protection against diphtheria, tetanus, polio, whooping cough, measles, mumps, rubella, and hepatitis B, as well as infections by meningococcus C, pneumococcus, and *Hemophilus influenzae* type B. Faced with the rise in cases of measles and whooping cough linked to the increasing number of unvaccinated children, some governments, like those of Australia and Germany, have made these vaccinations mandatory for registration in daycare or school. More recently, Austria became the first country to impose vaccination against COVID-19.

Vaccines are drugs that are—in the vast majority of cases—used to prevent diseases. The mistrust of vaccines that we observe today is a warning about the possible rejection, in the decades to come, of future preventive drugs that will be designed and developed thanks to AI, regardless of their effectiveness and their safety…

Innovation, Precaution, Transparency, and Education

We have previously discussed the economic aspect of technological innovation that supports a knowledge economy and generates considerable wealth. However, each technological breakthrough can induce significant ethical and societal problems. It is therefore crucial to adequately frame the development and use of new

[8] No cause-and-effect relationship between the MMR vaccination and autism could be demonstrated in large-scale studies conducted in response to this initial alert. On the other hand, all these clinical studies have unequivocally confirmed the effectiveness of the combined MMR vaccine against these three viral diseases, confirming a very favorable benefit/risk ratio.

technologies. This issue is reflected in the precautionary principle, which aims to take into consideration the potential risks of uncertain and irreversible damage linked to human activities. Initially, this principle invited putting in place proportional measures to prevent the theoretical risks associated with the introduction of new technologies, products, and substances. If the introduction of precautionary measures before risks manifest seems legitimate, the whole debate revolves around the "proportional" nature of these measures. Today, this precautionary principle is considered an indispensable protective wall for some but rather an inappropriate brake on innovation for others.

It is indeed essential to preserve technological innovation, with the assumption that, in a properly framed use, the expected benefits will far outweigh the risks incurred. From this perspective, more and more voices denounce the abusive use of the precautionary principle as a "conflict of disinterest" and advocate for replacing it with responsible innovation, as evoked by Hans Jonas under the term "*principle of responsibility*".[9] Concretely, responsible innovation involves the establishment of international rules that establish values to respect, good usage practices, and measures to prevent risks. These shared rules must ideally take into account the long-term effects of innovation on future generations. Obviously, establishing common rules at the international level can be difficult due to many divergent interests but also cultural differences between countries in the acceptance of technologies. For example, GMOs have sparked strong rejection in Europe when, at the same time, the controversy was more about the use of embryonic stem cells in the United States or animal experiments in Great Britain.

In this context, the European Union established in 2018 a principle of innovation in parallel with the precautionary principle in order to seek this balance that our contemporary societies must adopt when introducing new technologies.[10] By recommending that the impact on innovation of any new legislative initiative be evaluated, this principle invites consideration not only of potential health and environmental risks, as required by the precautionary principle, but also of the expected economic benefit. This recognition of technological innovation for competitiveness and economic development implicitly encourages measured risk-taking, assessable in light of societal benefits. We find here the concept of benefit-risk analysis encountered earlier in the evaluation by regulatory agencies of any new drug [3].

---

[9] Jonas [2]. In this essay at the origin of the concept of sustainable development, Hans Jonas emphasizes the responsibility of current generations in their decisions vis-à-vis future generations. French deputies recently refused to approve a bill that aimed to replace in the Constitution the precautionary principle by a principle of responsible innovation. This French posture is however far from being shared within the other countries of Europe.

[10] This concept has been particularly supported by the *European Risk Forum*, a think tank initially composed of industrial actors from the chemical, tobacco, and pesticide sectors, with the aim of proposing new risk management approaches to public authorities. This principle of innovation is mentioned in the introduction of the program *Horizon Europe*, launched by the European Commission in 2021, which allocates nearly 100 billion euros over 6 years to support research in Europe.

On the brink of an unprecedented wave of innovation driven by AI, in order to regain the public's trust in drugs, it will be necessary to openly share the rules that govern their development and use. It is also necessary for regulatory authorities, industry, and all drug stakeholders to communicate widely on the measures put in place to ensure the safety of drugs. This transparency in information and risk management is crucial to restore public trust in our postmodern democracies. More generally, the societal acceptance of applications from new technologies is a major issue for the twenty-first century. It will be just as vital to educate the public on these multidimensional subjects, to enlighten their opinion, and to avoid the spread of unfounded fears. If social networks are now a major source of information for young people, traditional media remain important for explaining complex scientific concepts to the general public. Therefore, it is also crucial to educate journalists and other actors involved in scientific popularization, as well as politicians, decision-makers, and funders.

For this purpose, scientists will need to get out of their laboratories to contribute to this massive education effort aimed at a wide audience. It is not only about explaining an issue but also about reporting on the rational approach that supports the scientific method envisaged to solve the problem. The controversy surrounding COVID-19 vaccines has shown that, on complex scientific subjects, not all opinions are to be considered at the same level. In an era where opinions can be easily manipulated, it is thus essential to restore the authority of scientific expertise. Realistically, this rehabilitation of rational thought and expertise appears today as a monumental task, as it faces a deep societal malaise. According to a recent poll, 82% of French people trust science, but only 68% trust scientists linked to the government, and 42% trust government representatives. This distrust of any authoritative speech associated with political power, also perceptible in many other countries, reflects a real democratic malaise, made visible by the rise of populist movements rejecting elites, including scientific experts.[11]

As demonstrated by the rejection of COVID-19 vaccines by a portion of the population, approaching facts rationally will inevitably clash with unfounded fears fueled by ignorance and perhaps even manipulation of opinion. The new drug intelligence at the center of this book is part of the assertion that scientific rationality remains the preeminent method for understanding the world beyond simple descriptions of phenomena. Thus, to act with discernment in order to transform it for the better by placing the human being at the center of all concerns.

[11] Survey conducted in October 2021 by IPSOS. Another recent survey conducted in France indicates that 48% of French people believe that scientific progress brings more good than harm to society, but 41% lean towards as much good as harm. See also the article by L. Rouban, Polytechniques Insights. *La defiance de la science n'est qu'une traduction du malaise démocratique.* February 9, 2022.

References

1. Brisson M, et al. Impact of HPV vaccination and cervical screening on cervical cancer elimination: a comparative modelling analysis in 78 low-income and lower-middle income countries. Lancet. 2020;395:575.
2. Jonas H. The imperative of responsibility: in search of an ethics for the technological age. Chicago: University of Chicago Press; 1985.
3. Benefit-risk assessment for new drug and biological products guidance for industry. Draft guidance, September 2021. https://www.fda.gov/media/152544

14 Priority to the Human

The Centaur Theory, or the Synergy of Intelligences

In the twentieth century, interactions between humans and intelligent machines will be daily and multiple. As previously mentioned, it is even likely that these interactions will take the form of hybridizations between human bodies and machines. For the future of our species, it is important that the convergence between human intelligence and artificial intelligence is successful. To understand its interest, including in the field of health, let's take a brief detour toward intelligent games.

For the general public, the spectacular performances of machines in these games have probably been the first concrete manifestation of the advances in AI. Many games indeed offer a multitude of choices and actions that require remarkable abilities in terms of reasoning, strategy, and anticipation, which we thought were reserved for our species. However, machines have seriously questioned the superiority of human intelligence in this playground.[1] The first competitions between human champions and computers began in the middle of the twentieth century, with very simple games, like checkers. In 1979, an algorithm beat a world champion for the first time, in this case in backgammon. In 1997, IBM's Deep Blue machine beat the world chess champion Garry Kasparov. A step had been taken, given the notorious complexity of chess in terms of the diversity of situations and possible moves. At the beginning of the twenty-first century, advances accelerated, demonstrating that AI could now surpass humans in most games, among the most sophisticated.

[1] Some definitions of intelligence encompass the ability to play complex games. Ironically, these advances of machines are primarily the fruit of human intelligence, that of scientists and engineers who have created machines capable of rivaling, or even surpassing human intelligence in this field, as in many others.

P. Moingeon, *Intelligent Drugs: How AI is Transforming Healthcare*, https://doi.org/10.1007/978-3-031-91668-7_14

Thus, in 2016, DeepMind's AlphaGo program beat South Korean Go world champion Lee Sedol by a score of 4 games to 1. To understand the scope of this success, remember that the game of Go involves placing white and black stones on a grid with the aim of conquering territories by encircling the opponent's stones. All pieces have the same value, but the possibilities of play are practically infinite. The number of possible configurations in a game is estimated at 10^{170} (the number 10 followed by 169 zeros!), which is more than the number of atoms in the universe! What makes AlphaGo exceptional is that it does not just execute predefined game systems. Of course, the software was trained using deep learning to reproduce the movements of the best players, memorizing more than 30 million games played by experts for this purpose. But AlphaGo also improved by continuously playing against itself, which is called reinforcement learning. This dual learning method allows AlphaGo to interpret the strategies of the opponent and to propose, in response, the best possible moves, without being able to explain its choice. While a professional Go player can anticipate up to 20 moves in advance, it is estimated that AlphaGo can consider all possible scenarios up to 60 moves in advance!

Is our species then destined to be inevitably surpassed by machines in the face-off between human and artificial intelligence? The answer is no, for several reasons. First of all, games are only a specific domain of human intelligence. Although machines can currently surpass humans in defined tasks for which they have been programmed, they are currently unable to excel in several areas at the same time or to perform optimally on unexpected problems. Moreover, a very valuable lesson learned from these confrontations in intelligent games is that human champions can also significantly improve by training with machines! In fact, they even start to win against them again, adopting their strategies and secret weapons.

This state of affairs in games foreshadows a fascinating future in all areas: that of a synergy between human and artificial intelligence, known as the centaur theory (see Box 14.1).

Box 14.1: The Centaur Theory or the Convergence of Intelligences

The word centaur refers to a mythological animal, half-man, half-horse. It could refer in the course of the twenty-first century to the hybrid intelligence resulting from the encounter between the human brain and the computer. This idea was born following the defeat in 1997 of chess champion Gary Kasparov during his confrontation with IBM's Deep Blue program. After initially being completely disheartened, Kasparov quickly understood his interest in what he called *centaur chess*, that is to say, the practice of a chess game "in centaur mode," consisting of training with the machine to progress in his discipline. This model of cooperation between humans and the intelligent machine is obviously not limited to intelligent games. It applies to all areas where modeling reality from existing data and knowledge is useful to make the best decisions.

(continued)

Box 14.1 (continued)

The underlying reason is simple: humans and intelligent machines approach problems in a different and complementary way. Human beings represent physical reality from their knowledge to build their reasoning, which they translate into hypotheses. In this respect, they can be biased by the assumptions and determinism acquired from their current psychological and emotional state, their experience, and their education. But they also bring intuition and imagination, dimensions absent in machines.

The machine brings its memory capacity, as well as its power and speed of calculation, which allow it to analyze massive amounts of data. The intelligent machine models the data by establishing, without a priori, a predictive mathematical algorithm that often appears to the human as a black box. Even if the machine is not exempt from bias, especially those related to data provided by humans, it considerably broadens the scope of the analysis beyond preconceived ideas and current knowledge, thus proposing solutions beyond the framework familiar to humans.

The artificial neural networks used in artificial intelligence do not function exactly like the human brain, the latter relying not only on synaptic connections between neurons but also on interactions between entire areas of the brain organized in modules. This remarkably connected organization makes the human brain particularly efficient. It is estimated that if a human brain could mobilize all its neurons at the same time on a single task, no existing computer would be as powerful! What's more, human intelligence consumes much less energy than an intelligent machine! Thus, during the Go game between the AlphaGo software and Lee Sedol, the machine consumed 1500 kW of energy when only 20 W were used by the human champion!

Machines develop efficient algorithms by analyzing large amounts of data. On the other hand, human intelligence learns by observation and by analyzing the consequences of actions performed or imagined, thus being aware of its successes and mistakes, which allows it to learn lessons to improve its performance. The machine calculates, and the human being reasons. Even if machines surpass humans in calculation, correlation, and classification, they are not endowed with thought. They therefore struggle to establish cause-and-effect links, hence the often unexplained nature of their conclusions. Not being embodied, machines will never be able to feel human emotions and feelings, nor will they manifest a true consciousness or intentionality.

Therefore, it is in standardized and automatable tasks—for example, the analysis of medical images—that intelligent machines are beginning to supplant humans. However, in these same tasks, human and artificial intelligence remain complementary. When an artificial neural network detects a tumor in an image, the machine provides a result without explaining the underlying reasoning, unlike human thought, which will justify its diagnosis on the basis of the morphological characteristics of the tissues and cells. Although efforts are underway to make algorithms more interpretable, their current lack of transparency contrasts with human thought capable of detailing the process leading to an idea or decision.[2]

Artificial intelligence allows for modeling based on mathematical logic, which admirably complements the reasoned but also subjective and intuitive approach of the human being to apprehend the complexity of the world. Another crucial complementarity lies in the fact that, while machines provide unparalleled computing power—and therefore analysis—humans are the guarantors of the rules and ethics that must guide the applications that result from it. A positive use of AI, therefore, requires successful convergence between human and artificial intelligence. Just like in games, this combination of human and machine skills will help humans make decisions and take informed action in the real world in the coming decades.

This synergy is also valid in the world of medicine and, more generally, in health. In this new ecosystem, traditional innovation players will need to develop skills in AI and digital technologies. Like chess or Go players, researchers and all health professionals will undoubtedly learn a lot from their interactions with intelligent machines. However, many scientists today are very wary of AI, worried about being dispossessed of their expertise by machines called to supplement them, or even replace them, in an increasing number of tasks. A key issue, therefore, is the necessary acculturation of human experts to these new technologies so that they become a source of new opportunities rather than a threat. Training in new technologies, not only for students but also for researchers and confirmed health professionals, is imperative so that they can consider how to use these new technologies to reduce their tedious tasks and create new possibilities in their fields of activity while maintaining a critical mind on their limits.

In human-intelligent machine interactions, another challenge will be to define the residual responsibilities of human experts. Human expertise will be essential in the selection and validation of data provided to the machine, as well as its use in compliance with regulations and ethics. In the decades to come, health professionals will remain responsible for decisions that concern the diagnosis of diseases, the determination of health risks, and the prescription and dispensation of medicines, even though these will increasingly rely on an AI solution. This human responsibility will persist until the emergence of truly autonomous machines, whose reliability of predictive algorithms will be firmly established.

Protecting Personal Data

The AI applications mentioned above are made possible by an abundance of available data. Today, humanity generates colossal quantities, as we have seen on the zettabyte scale (10^{21} bytes). More than 90% of these data are in the form of images,

[2] In the case of medical image analysis, it is now possible to identify attention mechanisms, to make the AI "say" which part of the image it used to classify a tumor or a tissue lesion.

texts, and messages exchanged by email or on social networks. These "unstructured" data are not formatted to be used by traditional computer tools, but with AI, they are now exploitable. We have highlighted the interest of digital technologies in the collection, storage, sharing, and dematerialized analysis of vast quantities of health data on a population scale. These combined advances now allow us to exploit not only the data accumulated by hospitals and city practitioners but also those produced by biomedical research in laboratories or during clinical studies evaluating new drugs. In the future, molecular profiling technologies, imaging, diagnostics, sensors, and connected objects will generate even more health data, not only concerning patients but also healthy individuals. The valorization of these massive data is today identified as an essential driver of medical innovation, notably by effectively developing new diagnostics and innovative drugs.

Aware of the economic value of these *big data*, developed countries have recently implemented policies to better exploit these resources, which were hitherto neglected. However, health data are not like other data; they become particularly sensitive when they concern a risk or a diagnosis of a serious disease, HIV seropositivity, or an addictive behavior. The confidentiality of these personal data is therefore crucial to avoid all kinds of societal, economic, or even political discrimination.

In parallel, other questions arise: Who owns these data? How to store them safely from hacking? How to control their diffusion?[3] Currently, the massive storage and sharing of data are managed by cloud computing, which replaces storage on a specific server. The technology of the blockchain, designed in 2008 for cryptocurrency exchanges, is another option to ensure the secure storage and transmission of health data. The blockchain is particularly interesting to the pharmaceutical industry for exploiting clinical trial data but also for tracing the origin of drugs to fight against their counterfeiting. As a manifestation of the newly recognized value of health data, some platforms on the blockchain, including that of the American company Longenesis, now allow individuals to monetize the sequence of their genome in exchange for compensation in cryptocurrencies.

The protection of personal data is essential, as demonstrated in 2016 by the Facebook case. Facebook made available to the company Cambridge Analytica, the data of millions of its customers then used to influence the American elections and the vote on Brexit. Well beyond this scandal, other examples already illustrate the extent of the problem, including in the field of health. A recent study of more than 200 digital health applications showed that more than 80% of these applications, particularly those used for tracking patients with diabetes, do not sufficiently

[3] Some warn of the risk that health data could be used by insurers to evaluate behaviors, in a perspective of bonus-malus linked to the health risks incurred. A European *think tank*, the *Digital New Deal Foundation*, advocates for responsible and humanistic (sic) data management in Europe, which preserves the interests of the individual.

protect private data.[4] Until recently, American legislation, which was less restrictive than that in Europe, allowed private companies like DeepMind to access the medical and genomic databases of patients through partnerships with public health or health insurance organizations.[5] Faced with the affirmed interest of the American digital giants GAFAM and Chinese BATHX in the private data of millions of people, with insufficient control over their use or dissemination, legitimate concerns are being raised. While some countries advocate the free use of personal data, others recommend strictly regulated access and sharing, with the implementation of a concerted international regulation of the type of expanded GDPR (see Box 14.2).

Box 14.2: General Regulation on Data Protection in Europe

In 2018, Europe was a pioneer in this field by promoting a responsible approach in the use of data to accompany the digital revolution. To this end, Europe has established rules to manage the access, dissemination, and use of personal data. This regulation, harmonized within the countries of the European Union, is called the GDPR (or General Data Protection Regulation).

The European GDPR highlights the notion of sensitive personal data, such as personal opinions, ethnic origins, as well as genetic or biometric data. It requires the informed consent of individuals for the use of their data for a specific purpose, as well as their anonymization to preserve confidentiality. It establishes security criteria, storage duration, and restricted and controlled transfer of data to third parties, particularly outside Europe.

European countries have adapted the GDPR into their respective national laws by establishing strict rules for the preservation of digital files created by companies or administrations. These rules classically require data holders to obtain the consent of individuals to collect their personal information, to restrict their exploitation to specified purposes, to guarantee the security of these data, to allow their deletion, and to offer everyone the possibility to refuse profiling by automated algorithms.[6]

---

[4] Bates et al. [1] and Perakslis et al. [2]. These studies recommend increased regulation by the FDA in the USA to better guarantee the reliability and respect of private data, used today by more than 350,000 digital health applications for diagnostic aid or patient monitoring purposes.

[5] In 2016, the medical records of nearly two million patients with kidney diseases were transferred to Google DeepMind, with the commendable aim of improving patient monitoring. However, these patients had not been consulted for the sharing of their data with DeepMind, which had not made any commitment to guarantee their confidentiality.

[6] In case of non-compliance, companies risk heavy fines that can reach up to 4% of their global turnover.

Although Europe invests ten times less in digital technologies and AI than the United States or China, this ethical regulation in the use of data could eventually confer a competitive advantage to the old continent, a pioneer in the field. In the United States, the regulation on the subject is much less restrictive. The *Health Insurance Portability and Accountability Act* (HIPAA) was established in 1996 to protect individual health data while allowing its dissemination and use for the proper functioning of the health system and public health policies. At a time when the GDPR is being deployed in Europe, there is no harmonized regulation at the international level regarding the use of personal data, even if, obviously, such an evolution in this direction is highly desirable.[7] A first colloquium entitled *Privacy International* was organized in 2019 to reflect in a concerted manner between countries on the issues of consent and sharing of health data. The subject will obviously remain topical in the years to come, given the recognized importance of data since AI allows it to extract its value, thus triggering a rush toward the new El Dorado of big data.

Another aspect related to the emergence of AI, particularly in health, is the question of the ownership of data and applications generated by AI from these data. As in other fields, intellectual property rules in the field of medicine are based on patents. With an AI capable of exploiting all types of data, intellectual property rules will need to be adapted. Research laboratories around the world have indeed started a frantic competition to create intellectual property from public data. The notion of inventiveness, essential for filing a patent, will be hotly debated in the case of an invention based on AI, on the grounds that it was implicitly contained in the data! The claim to the ownership of the data itself will be crucial, sparking fierce debates between the parties concerned, given the economic stakes. In the field of health, some patients and healthy individuals will be tempted to demand compensation for access to their health data for research purposes. The patentability of applications or even knowledge extracted by AI from health data will probably be the source of many legal disputes. These debates will not be without recalling some quarrels nearly 25 years ago around the patentability of knowledge about living things based on simple genome sequencing, finally prohibited. As a matter of fact, the regulation of AI uses in health can be inspired by some of the principles acquired during a previous major technological revolution, that of biotechnologies.[8]

---

[7] The Obama government has implemented legislation in the USA facilitating access to health data of American patients by digital giants, whose business model lies in the storage, sharing, and analysis of data. And this, in order to stimulate scientific research within the framework of the *Precision Medicine Initiative.*

[8] At the beginning of the third millennium, some laboratories began to patent genetic sequences whose function was unknown. This type of patent was eventually banned on the grounds that it concerns the heritage of humanity. In 2001, the European Parliament asked the European Patent Office to preserve "*the principle of non-patentability of human beings, their cells or genes in their natural environment*". This resolution led notably to the revocation of the patent of the company Myriad Genetics in Europe. This patent was about a method of diagnosing breast cancers based on knowledge of the human genome (focusing on the detection of mutations of the BRCA1 gene). It had been criticized in Europe for limiting access to this diagnosis and hindering innovation, thus opposing the public interest.

The Ethics of AI Inspired by Biotechnologies

The popularization of a new form of generative AI, with ChatGPT, led in March 2023 to calls for a moratorium on research in this field, in a letter signed by hundreds of scientists and personalities, including Elon Musk and other tech enthusiasts, who were previously unconditional supporters of AI. This particularly alarmist text questions the possibilities of using conversational agents of the GPT-4 type to the detriment of humanity, but also the speed of the evolution of the technologies that make up AI, even suggesting a potential existential risk for our species in case of the emergence of an uncontrolled superintelligence.

In consideration of these legitimate questions about the future properties of AI, but also in order to promote its beneficial applications, notably in health, a legal and ethical framework is now necessary. While the legal sphere aims to regulate by law, ethical reflection, which integrates human concern, is interested in the distinction between good and evil, beyond legal obligations. In particular, ethics questions the long-term consequences, especially important in the field of AI, and can, in this respect, guide the creation of laws and standards to prevent anticipated risks.

In order to establish these rules that will guide the applications of intelligent machines and, more generally, their interactions with humans, several elements must be considered. Ethics evolves with knowledge and experience; however, it does so on a longer time scale than that of technological progress. Moreover, the legal and ethical framework should concern not only the control of machines but also of humans. Beyond the risks that will be associated with the emergence of increasingly autonomous intelligent machines, it is indeed in the short term the inappropriate, criminal, or malicious human uses that must be avoided. Moreover, given the many expected benefits of using AI in health, as in many other fields, regulations should not prevent innovation for the benefit of humanity. The United States and China, joined by France and Germany, have thus recently alerted the European bodies to the fact that the *European AI Act*, initially envisaged by the European Commission, could constitute an obstacle to innovation, with disastrous economic consequences.

Regulating AI ideally requires agreement at the international level on ethical principles reflecting a universal vision of the individual and collective rights of the human being, which are essential to protect. A trustworthy AI requires the establishment of rules that govern the purposes, for example, in the programming of intelligent machines, so that they integrate and serve human needs. Shared standards at the global level are highly desirable in the form of good usage practices that ensure, on the one hand, the transparency and explainability of algorithms and, on the other hand, inclusivity by controlling the biases of algorithms or those introduced in the data used.

Although these requirements seem very ambitious, there are reasons to be optimistic. A particularly interesting reference concerns the concerted regulation at the global level that has successfully accompanied the revolution of biotechnologies over the last 40 years. In the 1980s, the emergence of technologies allowing the manipulation of living organisms by the transfer of genetic material raised many ethical questions. It then became urgent to regulate these developments to avoid harmful consequences while continuing to explore the potential benefits for humanity, particularly in the field of health. A few decades later, thanks to proportionate and evolving regulation, a major revolution was able to take place with the sequencing of the human genome, gene therapy, and hundreds of biological drugs and immunotherapies, transforming the lives of billions of patients. Without biotechnologies, we would not have effective vaccines today to control the COVID-19 pandemic and allow humanity to resume a normal life.

Importantly, the example of biotechnologies has shown that at a first level, the scientific community is capable of self-regulation (see Box 14.3).

Box 14.3: From One Asilomar to Another

An effective means of regulation by the scientific community is to define strict rules for controlling research activities in a new field while waiting to clarify the issues and implications. These commonly accepted rules can go as far as a moratorium, that is, the temporary suspension of these activities. The most emblematic example of self-regulation in the scientific field is that of the Asilomar conference, which brought together in 1975 in California 150 researchers from around the world working on genetic manipulations. The central question was about the risks of genetic modification of the bacterium *Escherichia coli* to make it produce proteins of interest from animal or human genes. This technology, perfectly mastered today, is at the basis of the production of many therapeutic proteins called "recombinant proteins" used as drugs to treat cancers or inflammatory diseases.

This moratorium on genetic manipulations has sometimes been criticized for overestimating the risks—ultimately unproven—of DNA recombination technology in creating biological organisms that are dangerous to humanity. This prompted the NIH (*National Institutes of Health*, Bethesda, USA) to issue recommendations on biosafety, which, according to some researchers, delayed scientific progress by several years. On a positive note, however, it has promoted a gradual acceptance of advances in the field of life technologies by establishing common rules. Asilomar also demonstrated the need to regularly update the regulatory framework for new technologies, as their impact and associated risks were better understood.

In January 2017, a similar meeting was organized again at Asilomar, bringing together experts in artificial intelligence to establish recommendations for the scientific community working in this field. Initial general principles were issued to accompany the development of AI, make it more transparent, and ensure its use for the benefit of humanity. These principles concern the regulation of research, respect for ethical values, and the risks to be considered in the short or long term.[9]

[9] See Tegmark [3]. Also see http://futureoflife.org/ai-principles

Since the first Asilomar of 1975, experts from different fields in the life sciences have continued to meet regularly to refine ethical and practical rules, which are shared later within the scientific community at the global level. In recent years, researchers have proposed the creation of "ethical zones" in biology that should not be explored, even if the technologies allow it. These concerns, for example, include the engineering of bacteria to produce illegal drugs or the creation of potentially dangerous infectious agents, such as modified flu viruses. In 2019, scientists proposed a moratorium in the journal *Nature* in response to the unauthorized work of Chinese researcher He Jiankui, who genetically modified human embryos with CRISPR-Cas9 technology.[10]

In addition to this self-regulation, the experience of biotechnologies has also shown the importance of involving other actors, beyond researchers, to design bioethics laws. These have been implemented in many countries, relying on independent multidisciplinary committees capable of examining not only the technical and scientific dimensions but also the sociological, philosophical, economic, and environmental implications related to these new technologies. Their recommendations have helped to understand the complexity and uncertainties related to the potential impacts of these advances, contributing to establishing a framework at the national level for the manipulation of living beings and the applications of biotechnologies. These recommendations have then been regularly updated as knowledge progresses. In France, the first law on bioethics was established in 1994, then updated successively in 2014, 2011, and 2021, relying on extensive public consultations, particularly useful for better informing and educating citizens on a large scale. Moreover, the field of biotechnologies has shown that it is possible to harmonize positions between countries. Although there are still differences, international regulations have indeed been established on several subjects, such as the regulated manipulation of embryos for research purposes or the prohibition of human cloning.[11]

In total, the legal and ethical framework for biotechnologies, based on an evolving benefit-risk assessment, has allowed for extraordinarily beneficial innovation for humanity. It can inspire the regulation of applications of artificial intelligence in health, moreover, in synergy with life technologies. Recently, regulations have been put in place in the European community—also a pioneer in this field at the global level—to regulate the applications of AI. In particular, the final version of the European AI Act, adopted by the European Parliament on December 8, 2023, aims to establish a responsible AI that puts the human at the center while not hindering innovation. The text clarifies the definition of artificial intelligence systems, which include autonomous AI or AI implanted on a device. It prohibits uses contrary to the charter of fundamental rights in terms of cognitive or behavioral manipulation,

[10] Movements such as the *Responsive Science project* now invite researchers working on approaches to *gene editing* to openly share in advance their ideas and their experiment plans with the scientific community. This voluntary transparency approach allows researchers to gather advice from the scientific community before carrying out their laboratory experiments.

[11] The current international consensus is to prohibit the genetic manipulation of human germ cells, as well as their use to modify embryos with the aim of creating a genetically modified human being.

establishment of a social score, or remote biometric identification. The risks related to AI are addressed in this document according to different sectors of activity, with health being considered as carrying specific risks in terms of respect for privacy and intellectual property rights. The new European regulation also highlights the importance of information on how the AI solution was developed, as well as on its operation and the data used. It also recalls the responsibility of the AI provider but also that of the user, in compliance with its intended use.

To respect innovation, the European AI Act recommends flexible frameworks, in the form of regulatory sandboxes, to be able to experiment with new products, services, or activities. In addition to the GDPR mentioned above, the European AI Act encourages the use and increased sharing of data to enable an economy based on the use of these big data while ensuring personal data protection. In the health sector, the creation of a European health data space is envisaged, inspired by the French Health Data Hub, to facilitate the exploitation and secondary reuse of health data, particularly for biomedical research purposes.

Specifically, regarding generative AI, the text adopted in Europe requires ensuring the quality of the data used to train the algorithms, in compliance with any copyrights. Users must also specify that the texts, images, and music are produced with the help of AI. Beyond the European AI Act and the GDPR, the Digital Market Act further regulates competition rights, particularly for digital giants and access providers. The Digital Service Act also aims to hold platforms accountable for the dissemination of illegal content. The prescriptions of the European AI Act and all aforementioned regulations are being progressively enforced in various European countries since February 2025.

References

1. Bates D, et al. Health apps and health policy. What is needed? JAMA. 2018;320:1975.
2. Perakslis E, et al. Digital health, the need to assess benefits, risks and value. JAMA. 2021;325:127.
3. Tegmark M. Life 3.0. London: Penguin Books; 2017.

Epilogue

In December 2024, as I finished writing this book, by a happy coincidence, I participated in a thesis jury evaluating the work of Raphaelle, a young doctoral student in pharmacy, on the contributions of AI in oncology. This convincing work methodically and clearly lists the many applications of AI to assist in the diagnosis, treatment, and follow-up of patients with breast cancer. The jury members awarded the coveted degree to the young student. In a solemn moment filled with emotion, she swears with conviction to use all her knowledge for the benefit of the patients.

Young people who decide today to pursue a career in healthcare will have this unique opportunity in their professional life to be part of the revolution induced by AI. This upheaval also concerns established health professionals, researchers from academic laboratories, hospital staff, and employees of the pharmaceutical industry who have already been committed for years to helping those who suffer. The general public has not been mistaken, who applauded the courage and determination of caregivers in the fight against COVID-19, when the outcome was still uncertain. All these present and future health actors now have in their hands this extraordinary Promethean power conferred by the synergy between AI, biotechnologies, and drug sciences. This comes with the responsibility to ensure that these technologies are used for the common good.

If this is the case, the prospects are very exciting. Over the next 30 years, the knowledge of the uniqueness of each individual—sick or healthy—of their genetic or epigenetic risks will make medicine increasingly personalized and predictive. The role and responsibility of each person in managing their health will be magnified. Thanks to AI, many intelligent drugs will be developed, some preventing diseases, others treating rare diseases, increasing body performance, improving cognitive abilities, or slowing down aging.

All these upcoming changes are vast and must be approached with the human being as the primary concern. They require a profound overhaul of protection systems to handle this future wave of intelligent drugs. Health actors will need to train in AI to achieve the convergence of human and artificial intelligences. It will be essential to protect the patient's personal data while developing an AI ethic respectful of humans to enlighten all applications of these scientific and technological advances.

P. Moingeon, *Intelligent Drugs: How AI is Transforming Healthcare*,
https://doi.org/10.1007/978-3-031-91668-7

Clearly, individual and societal representations of humanity will evolve over the century in light of numerous and sophisticated interfaces with intelligent machines. Undoubtedly, the revolution brought by intelligent drugs will play a significant role in the technological evolution of humankind in the twenty-first century.

MIX
Papier aus verantwortungsvollen Quellen
Paper from responsible sources
FSC® C105338

If you have any concerns about our products,
you can contact us on
ProductSafety@springernature.com

In case Publisher is established outside the EU,
the EU authorized representative is:
Springer Nature Customer Service Center GmbH
Europaplatz 3, 69115 Heidelberg, Germany

Printed by Libri Plureos GmbH
in Hamburg, Germany